ITSY BITSY
Yoga

Poses to Help Your Baby
Sleep Longer, Digest Better,
and Grow Stronger

● ● ●

Helen Garabedian

A FIRESIDE BOOK
Published by Simon & Schuster
New York   London   Toronto   Sydney

FIRESIDE
Rockefeller Center
1230 Avenue of the Americas
New York, NY 10020

For information regarding special discounts for bulk purchases,
please contact Simon & Schuster Special Sales at 1-800-456-6798
or business@simonandschuster.com

Designed by Jaime Putorti

Manufactured in the United States of America

10   9   8   7   6   5   4   3   2   1

Library of Congress Cataloging-in-Publication Data
Garabedian, Helen.
  Itsy bitsy yoga : poses to help your baby sleep longer, digest better, and grow stronger /
Helen Garabedian
    p. cm.
  "A Fireside Book."
  1. Hatha yoga for infants. 2. Infants—Health and hygeine. 3. Parent and infant. I. Title
RJ133.7 .G37 2004
649'.122—dc22
2004041638

ISBN 0-7432-4355-2

Acknowledgments

. . . .

My profound gratitude goes to my students, teachers, and the babies who inspire me with wisdom, creativity, and direction.

I would also like to acknowledge and give thanks to:

- My dear husband, David, for his patience, love, and understanding.
- My entire family, especially my Mother, who raised me so lovingly and cultivated my spirituality and practice of yoga.
- My childhood friend, Kelly Rainho, for helping keep the child in me alive and playing.
- Patricia Burke for her undying support, kindness, and guidance.
- Earthsong Yoga Center in Marlboro, Massachusetts, for becoming the birthplace of Itsy Bitsy Yoga.
- Bonnie Bainbridge Cohen and the teaching staff at The School for Body-Mind Centering for being luminaries in the field of Infant Developmental Movement Education.
- Dr. Harvey Karp and Julie Carson May of the Happiest Baby Inc. for being champions in the lives of parents and babies.
- Kristie Babbin for believing in me and managing all the families who have shared themselves in photographs.
- All the Certified Itsy Bitsy Yoga facilitators who bring parents, babies, and toddlers together for classes.

Finally, I am grateful for the people who helped me manifest this book. They include my ambitious literary agent, Carol Susan Roth; Lisa Considine, who saw the potential of my work; Cherise Davis, senior editor at Fireside/Simon & Schuster, who is simply one of the best; and the entire staff at Fireside for their ongoing support.

Contents

• • • • • • • • • • •

Introduction

· · · · · · · · · · · · · · · ·

A baby's most natural state is bliss. Open, curious, and content, babies are designed to give and receive love. However, sometimes a baby's true state falls a little off kilter and needs help to rebalance. Since babies do not come with instruction manuals, I teach parents and caregivers simple yoga-based movements and techniques to help free babies from suffering from digestion troubles and liberate their restlessness into peaceful sleep and happiness. You, as the caregiver, don't need any yoga experience to calm your baby and help him or her grow strong. All you need to do is breathe, love, and move!

What Is Yoga?

The word *yoga* has acquired many translations over the centuries. According to *The Heart of Yoga,* by T. K. V. Desikachar, meanings of the word include "to unite," "to come together," "to tie the strands of the mind together," and "acting in such a way that all of our attention is directed toward the activity in which we are currently engaged." Yoga gives us insight. The practice of yoga with a baby can help parents and caregivers bond with the baby more deeply, and understand how best to care for them. When parents come to my yoga studio, they are not distracted by the outside world. Yoga can bring moms and dads closer to understanding and supporting their child's intentions, needs, and desires. Through yoga, babies sense their parents' trust and deep commitment to understanding and responsiveness as they move forward in developing their physical, social, intellectual, and emotional skills in the way that is aligned with each child's highest destiny.

What Is Itsy Bitsy Yoga®?

Itsy Bitsy Yoga is a unique blend of yoga postures, infant developmental movement, and parent/child bonding. In this book, you will find nearly seventy easy-to-learn and practical poses and techniques that benefit your child from birth to twenty-four months old. I have intertwined the cross-cultural jewels from the wisdom of an infant's moving body, yoga, and the latest research in the field of infant development to deliver a developmentally nutritious movement program for a parent and baby to enjoy together.

In teaching yoga to facilitators and thousands of babies, toddlers, and parents, I have seen firsthand the benefits of yoga for babies: better sleep, improved digestion, relief from gas pains and mild colic, a stronger immune system, and an increase in body awareness and self-confidence.

The Birth of Itsy Bitsy Yoga

As a certified yoga teacher and infant developmental movement educator, I examine Hatha Yoga postures with the intention of adapting them for the nonverbal baby to do with or without a parent's help. The culmination of my professional background, twenty years of yoga and meditation practice, and a lifetime of study and experience in caring for babies and toddlers, is evident in Itsy Bitsy Yoga. Itsy Bitsy Yoga teaches parents how to support their baby's physical development and movement as nature intended. As much as possible I will tell you the role yoga plays in your child's development so that the experience and rewards are richer for you.

Not everything in this book is yoga in a traditional sense. I also translate the movements of an infant's natural developmental progression into playful practices. Many of my students are especially impressed that my poses and techniques are able to calm their babies so well.

I will show you how certain positions play a necessary role in your baby's physical development. I'll help you support your baby's physical development and the natural flow of unfolding gross motor skills. Lack of awareness in positioning, holding, or moving an infant can result in future lower back problems, reading difficulties, and challenges in focus.

The History of Baby Yoga

It is my belief that over thousands of years ago when yoga was first developing, yoga masters studied the movements of babies to create postures, or *asanas*. Through the practice of yoga, adults are returning to the unrestricted innocence and bliss of infancy. In a sense, yoga for babies has always existed. It is part of what babies do naturally. However, the natural movement babies need to experience is being reduced with the overuse of confining baby-holding devices such as infant car seats, walkers, seated activity centers, and strollers.

Yoga Is Natural for Babies

This photograph illustrates how an infant's development mirrors Classical Hatha Yoga postures developed more than five thousand years ago. For example, a baby coming up to a walking stance reflects the Downward Facing Dog Pose in Yoga.

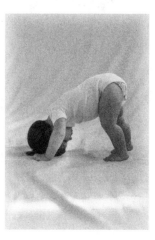

Baby in Downward Facing Dog Pose

Babies who are new to walking move into Downward Facing Dog repeatedly to transition from the floor into standing. Down Dog (as I like to call it in Itsy Bitsy Yoga) also occurs earlier in development when a baby is almost crawling. Throughout the book, I will explain what role Down Dog and other traditional Hatha Yoga postures play in your baby's development.

Top Five Reasons Why Babies Are Natural Yogis (yoga students)

1. Like yogis, babies prefer to breathe through the nose.
2. Like yogis, babies are only concerned with the present moment.
3. Like yogis, babies love unconditionally.
4. Like yogis, babies practice nonviolence.
5. Like yogis, babies practice yoga postures naturally as part of development.

Is It Too Early or Too Late for My Baby or Toddler to Start Yoga?

No. You're never too young or too old to start the practice of yoga. Parents and caregivers are invited to start practicing the postures in *Itsy Bitsy Yoga* with babies anytime between birth and twenty-four months. See Chapter 2 to get you started.

Yoga Takes as Little as Twenty Seconds and as Long as Twenty-five Minutes

The time you spend doing Itsy Bitsy Yoga is a vacation from the rest of your day. This developmentally nutritious activity also enhances your bond with your baby. A baby's or toddler's yoga practice can last twenty seconds to twenty-five minutes, depending on the baby's needs and your schedule. One of the book's nine Magic Poses (explained on page 10) can reduce fussiness almost instantaneously. In five to ten minutes you and your baby can engage in any one of the book's thirty-five Itsy Bitsy Yoga Series. Each series playfully combines three to seven postures to help you calm your baby, help your baby sleep longer, and grow stronger. Finally, you may choose to practice a number of the book's seventy yoga postures that are appropriate for your baby's current developmental stage.

No Yoga Experience Needed

No experience is necessary to share yoga and its benefits with a baby. Many people have always wanted to try yoga but thought they were too busy, until they became parents. In fact, more than half of the parents I teach had never done yoga before expecting a child. When a woman becomes pregnant she has more reason to pay attention to and care for her body in ways she might not have previously. Parents come to my classes to bond with and learn about their babies. After all, the word *yoga* means "to unite." When people learn how beneficial yoga is, they want to share it with their families. Also, my students have found yoga to be useful for enhancing the bond between a new baby and older siblings, grandparents, other family members, and nannies.

Molly and her fourteen-month-old son, Trevor, came to my class on a friend's referral. Molly had never tried yoga, but had known that someday she would like to. She thought it would be a good activity to share with her son, and it was! It turns out that Molly loved the time she spent practicing yoga with Trevor. Now, every time Trevor hears the words "Tree Pose," he assumes the Tree Pose in yoga! Molly has also begun practicing yoga for herself and finds that she has more energy to keep up with her growing toddler.

ITSY BITSY
Yoga

Chapter 1

How Yoga Can Help You and Your Baby

Top Twelve Reasons Why Babies and Toddlers Need Yoga

1. To help them sleep better and longer
2. To improve digestion and ease gas pain
3. To turn fussiness into happiness
4. To promote a healthy, physically fit lifestyle
5. To strengthen the parent-child bond
6. To increase neuromuscular development
7. To cultivate self-esteem and a positive body image
8. To boost the immune system
9. To reduce stress and develop relaxation techniques
10. To reduce anxiety
11. To increase body awareness
12. To aid the natural development of movement from birth to walking

The Benefits of Itsy Bitsy Yoga

For the baby/toddler participant, Itsy Bitsy Yoga can promote better sleep, improve digestion, ease gas pain and colic, stimulate neuromuscular development, and boost the immune system. Babies who have practiced Itsy

Bitsy Yoga appear to have greater body awareness and positive self-image as they grow into toddlers and preschoolers. Parents attribute these benefits to yoga.

Parents who practice Itsy Bitsy Yoga with their infants and toddlers notice a deeper parent-child bond, better sleep for everyone, and greater confidence in their parenting skills, which leads to less stress and anxiety. For repeat parents, Itsy Bitsy Yoga is also a special way to spend individual time with children born later in the birth order. By incorporating yoga into your baby's day, I am confident you will begin to notice the benefits I will discuss throughout this chapter.

Better and Longer Sleep

Nina, the mother of four-month-old Grace, planned to drive five hours to visit her family for a long weekend. Nina had noticed her baby took an extra long nap after practicing yoga, so she thought, "Perfect, we'll leave after our Itsy Bitsy Yoga class." And they did. Baby Grace slept and sat quietly without a fuss for the car ride from Massachusetts to New Jersey. At the end of the weekend, Nina packed and prepared to head home with Grace. It turned out that Nina had remembered everything except to practice baby yoga with her daughter before they left. Baby Grace cried and fussed for most of the drive home!

One of the reasons why Grace and other babies sleep better after yoga is because they are comfortable. Yoga engages muscles and then releases them, leaving a baby feeling content and relaxed. I've noticed that babies have longer, more restful naps after yoga practice. Parents also tell me that their babies wake less during the nights that follow Itsy Bitsy Yoga practice.

When you follow the poses in this book precisely, especially the Sleep Well Series, you may notice your baby beginning to sleep better and longer. If your baby does wake in the night, you can use Magic Poses (see page 10) to help calm your baby. Many parents have thanked me because Divine Drops (page 54) or another Sleep Well pose helped their baby go back to sleep with little effort. When yoga helps your baby sleep better, you'll get more sleep too! (Or at least you will once you get past the checking to make sure the baby's OK because he isn't waking up.)

Improved Digestion and Easing of Gas Pains

A newborn's intestines are sometimes paper thin. This makes digestion challenging. The developing digestive tissues of many babies require massage, yoga, or even dietary changes. For years, yoga has helped its adult practitioners digest by gently strengthening and massaging the intestines through body movement and positioning

Mom Eva was demonstrating to her husband, Jeff, how Apana Pose helped ten-week-old Jacob pass gas. Baby Jacob was on the changing table and diaperless when he passed more than just gas. Dad Jeff was impressed with yoga's effectiveness.

Observation and the time you spend helping your baby practice yoga will bring you a greater awareness of your baby's body and its movements. As you notice your baby's cues of digestive difficulty, you can assist and comfort her with the poses I present. In this book, I have indicated specific yoga poses that can help to rid your baby of abdominal gas and constipation.

Relief from Fussiness and Colic

I have named the practical techniques and poses that calm crying or fussy babies "Magic Poses." And they do work magic. Many times, these poses can calm a crying or fussy baby almost instantaneously. When practiced properly, Magic Poses transform the fussiest babies into the happiest babies. For a complete list of Magic Poses, see page 236.

I got a call from Susie, who was exhausted from trying various ways to calm Dylan, her colicky son. I offered to come over to Susie's house to show her and Dylan some Itsy Bitsy Yoga postures. This helped them both turn a huge corner. Divine Drops, a Magic Pose, repeatedly worked in calming Dylan. Susie even discovered that she could do Divine Drops on a big plastic yoga ball when she was tired or needed to relax. Itsy Bitsy Yoga gave Susie ways to calm her very fussy baby.

A Healthy, Physically Fit Lifestyle

Babies spend their days eating, sleeping, and figuring out how to move either themselves or toys. A baby's ability to move represents a level of physical wellness. Sharing structured and developmentally sound physical activities such as yoga, with infants, balances the time they are confined in strollers, playpens, car seats, and walkers. By devoting time to positively supporting a child's structured physical activities, parents set the foundation for a physically active childhood and beyond. Confined and sedentary infants or toddlers can grow to be sedentary children, leading to a vicious cycle of inactivity. Itsy Bitsy Yoga is designed in accordance with the physical activity guidelines for children birth to five years established by National Association for Sport and Physical Education. Yoga can easily become one of the structured physical activities that you choose to share with your infant and toddler.

Strengthened Bonds Between Parent and Child

Itsy Bitsy Yoga gives you a new way to bond with your baby. According to researcher Allan Schore, the bond between parent and baby in the first eighteen months after birth is the emotional foundation of all future bonding. Bonding offers parents the opportunity to witness and support their child's physical and emotional development.

During yoga the parent or caregiver and baby are able to step away from any distractions and focus on learning about each other. You and your baby can bond through many of the senses—touch, smell, sight, sound—and also through the biological rhythm of breathing. In Itsy Bitsy Yoga you can help make each child feel special as she senses, moves, and feels confident in her growing body!

Special Activity for Parent and Later-Born Children

Maria had a three-year-old son at home when I first met her and her daughter. Leah was six months old when they started yoga. Mom Maria found that doing yoga with Leah was the only time that she wasn't distracted by her other responsibilities. That one hour a week allowed priceless bonding and child-parent interaction for mother and daughter. Additionally, Maria became masterful at taking short yet frequent moments during her busy day to reconnect with Leah through yoga. Maria, now pregnant with her third baby, will continue find time to create bonds with her third child through yoga.

Neuromuscular Development

Did you know that during infancy the brain grows more than at any other time? Yes, it is true. An infant's brain at birth weighs a half a pound. By the first birthday, that brain has tripled to one and a half pounds. Stemming down from the brain are the spine and the neuromuscular system. Movement and touch help build neuromuscular pathways. Through repetitive movements these pathways are strengthened and the foundation for learning is built.

In Itsy Bitsy Yoga you will notice that repetitions are also important because they give your child the time recognize and to respond to the activity at hand. Through repetition, one-year-old Nolan has learned to crawl onto his mom's lap when I say the words "Hop Along Yogi" (one of his favorite yoga poses).

Self-Esteem and Positive Body Image

When you make time to practice yoga with your baby, you are cultivating self-esteem. Each baby deserves to feel she can become whatever her heart desires regardless of her life's circumstances. The one-on-one time yoga offers lets your baby know she is important and worthy of your attention. Many times these babies will grow up with a feeling of worthiness and confidence that leads to self-esteem.

For new parents, yoga helps cultivate self-esteem in parenting too! Jennifer started my program with her seven-week-old daughter, Olivia. Jennifer didn't have too much confidence in her parenting skills at the time. Initially, yoga helped her feel comfortable handling her baby. As our class continued Jennifer learned how to calm Olivia. She also learned Olivia's preferences and how to read her cues. Jennifer now has another baby whom she brings to class when Olivia, the big sister, is in preschool. Now, the newer parents in yoga class consider Jennifer to be a role model mom and look to her for advice.

Strengthened Immune System

Many hospitals now offer meditation, visualization, yoga, and other relaxation techniques to help boost the immune system and assist in fighting the effects of cancer and other serious illnesses. In fact, yoga can give the immune system help in preventing infections as it promotes overall detoxification. One pose that is particularly good at giving the immune system an added boost is Guppy Pose. Research shows that chronically high levels of stress hormones (like adrenaline) suppress the immune system and reduce the body's ability to defend or repair itself.

Stress, shameful negative experiences, and excessive scolding can depress one's immune system and harm self-esteem. When a baby is stressed his immune system is depleted and his ability to learn is diminished because of the focus on survival. When sharing yoga with babies we foster healthy, positive experiences with lots of praise. This will boost their immune systems and their self-esteem, making them stronger and healthier.

Reduced Stress

Studies show that children today encounter 25 percent more stress than their grandparents did. As parents, we need to realize the importance of stress-relieving activities such as yoga as vital for a child's well-being. It is never too early to offer your children tools to release the stressors of being a child today. Yoga triggers endorphins—the body's natural "feel good" hormones—which combat stress.

Some adults tend to find new situations stressful. Certainly parenting can be stressful for first-time parents. I have noticed that the parents who learn how to calm and understand their babies experience less stress than those who don't. Knowing how to calm your baby is like having a million dollars in a safe-deposit box: it is there when you need it. I will show you numerous poses to help calm both yourself and your baby.

Reduced Anxiety and Outside Stimulus

The stimulating demand our environment puts on babies is more excessive than in times past. Televisions, computers, electronic toys, videos— so many things can excite or stress a baby and say, "Check this out!" Babies are seldom given the opportunity to relax, and they tend to be kept as busy as their parents. Yoga teaches babies and adults how to experience relaxation and modulate their bodies into a quiet alert state. A child who can achieve a quiet alert state has good hormonal balance and will be focused and prepared to learn.

Baby yoga empowers parents and caregivers with the confidence and techniques needed to pull them through the more challenging days. I like to think of those as the days when your baby finds out what you're made of and just how much you care about his needs. Some parents feel anxious, responsible, or helpless when their baby is fussy, and that is unnecessary. A baby is not upset with anything a parent or caregiver has done. Babies are grateful and love you endlessly! Through yoga parents have a touchstone of wellness so their family can experience peace, love, and joy.

Some of the poses that I have developed, such as I Love You!, further teach babies how to modulate between opening up and reaching out into the world and then retreating back to their inner selves. The movement pattern of I Love You! is based on an inner and outer movement pattern that first takes place in fetal life. Retreating into one's center can be helpful for children with short attention spans or attention deficit disorder (ADD).

Increased Body Awareness

Babies can't read, write, or spell but they can move. Babies practice new positions and movement frequently as they develop and grow. Moving can be considered a baby's full-time job as she evolves from a newborn to walking within a relatively short time.

Babies whose movements are acknowledged and praised as good are apt to continue moving into a healthy, active lifestyle. A baby concludes, "People like the way I move," "Moving is good," and "I will continue to move my body." A moving baby and later a moving child are more likely to avoid a sedentary lifestyle and its associated emotional and physical problems.

Moving into yoga poses gives older babies a sense of accomplishment. Babies develop strong body awareness as they work toward achieving a yoga pose or movement with or without a loving adult's assistance. Sixteen-month-old Chloe will do Tree Pose for a quick moment before immediately smiling and clapping with joy at her accomplishment. Every child deserves a stage on which to showcase her talents and an audience to cheer her on.

Chapter 2

How to Use This Book

I believe that babies develop in their own unique way and time. For this reason I wrote this book based on developmental stages rather than ages. Start this book at anytime with your baby (from birth to twenty-four months of age) and it will be a wonderful experience. It is important for us to help children's abilities unfold without rushing them or wishing they could do something their bodies simply aren't ready for yet. It is important for a baby to learn to crawl. However, is not important for that baby to crawl by the age of eight months. Obviously, age-driven milestones are useful to a doctor charting a baby's progress but they are irrelevant in yoga. The importance in yoga is seeing and enjoying where a baby is in the present moment.

Yoga can be practiced in twenty seconds to twenty-five minutes. In this chapter, we will take a closer look at the various avenues you can take in sharing yoga with your baby. Magic Poses, Itsy Bitsy Yoga Series, the Bond & Be Well, and Quick Fix Techniques as well as the elements of the Developmentally Based Yoga chapters will be discussed as the Itsy Bitsy way of sharing yoga with your baby.

It Is Easy to Share Yoga Regularly!

TECHNIQUE	PRACTICE OPTIONS	DURATION	PURPOSE
Quick Fix Technique	Magic Pose Series	20 to 60 seconds	Make baby happy
Bond & Be Well Technique		5 to 10 minutes	Short, effective routines
	Chapter of Poses for current developmental stage	15 to 25 minutes	Learn postures' techniques and benefits

Magic Poses Can Stop Crying in Sixty Seconds or Less

Magic Poses incorporate developmental movement, cultural calming techniques, singing, and yoga. Originally, I created Magic Poses to draw wandering and mobile babies back into the yoga practice. But I've discovered my Magic Poses bring most babies happiness. You will too find Magic Poses turn a baby's fussiness into smiles. With yoga, you have a new tool to calm your baby in a short amount of time!

Magic Poses are easy to do anytime, even in the middle of the night. Magic Poses work best when they are done with the right intensity and when practiced regularly. I'll guide you in finding the right intensity, and with practice you will fine-tune it. In order for Magic Poses to work, your baby's needs for food and sleep must be met. Each chapter of yoga poses has a magic pose for you to use. The older your baby gets, the more Magic Poses you can choose from. But don't worry: Divine Drops, Swirlies, Apana, and the Happy Baby Series work great in the days and weeks after your baby's birth. Don't try to practice Magic Poses that your baby is not developmentally ready for. Practice only those that are appropriate for your baby at each stage. By the time a baby reaches age two, parents have nine Magic Poses to help their family. (For a complete list of Magic Poses, see page 236). Magic Poses are fun to practice and make calming your baby's cries much easier.

The Itsy Bitsy Yoga Poses Series

You've learned how good yoga can be for babies and toddlers, but like many parents you're probably asking, "When am I going to find the time?" To solve this problem I've created the Itsy Bitsy Yoga Poses Series. At the end of each developmentally based yoga chapter you will find the Good Morning Series, the Developmental Play Series, the Happy Baby Series, the Daddy Series, and the Sleep Well Series. Each series takes about five minutes and consists of three to seven poses specifically designed to address sleep, crying, bonding, development, or fun!

Good Morning Series

The Good Morning Series is for you to practice as soon as your baby wakes up, or anytime within the first hour. During the Good Morning Series keep outside stimulation to a minimum. Use the natural light of the day and leave the stereo and TV turned off. The Good Morning Series can also be practiced after your baby's nap.

Developmental Play Series

The Developmental Play Series gives you tools to help your baby grow strong physically and mentally. Let the Developmental Play Series give you a new way to see where your baby is today. Notice changes in his body's movements. What is he doing this week that he wasn't doing last week? Perhaps you'd like to note his physical development in a journal. It will make a nice keepsake for him someday and may be useful if you have more babies.

Happy Baby Series

The Happy Baby Series is designed to make your baby happy. Many of poses in the Happy Baby Series I created to supplement the traditional Hatha Yoga asanas I teach to new families. When the poses within this series are performed with the best velocity and rhythm for your baby, you'll notice your baby can shift from red-faced screaming to a joyful smile. The Happy Baby Series can be used when your baby is either sad or happy. If practiced when your baby is cheerful she will remain so, and may even become happier. If your baby is crying or fussy, the Happy Baby Series should change her tune to a happy one. Stick with the sequence of the series and hopefully you'll see a shift in your baby's state. The Happy Baby Series will not replace a baby's need for food, sleep, or cleanliness. All of your baby's basic survival needs must be met before you can expect the Happy Baby Series to help stop your baby from crying.

Daddy Series

Both parents provide for a child, but what they provide can be very different. Traditionally, dads are the more physical beings and moms the more emotional beings. It is a wonderful experience for your child to experience both of these qualities so that no matter the baby's gender they are balanced. Allow your baby the opportunity to embody a sense of what it is like to be to be physical and strong and free-loving and emotional with both parents. Your baby will experience yoga differently with different people. The presence of the adult, and the varying qualities of touch, velocity, breath, and rhythm all play into how your baby perceives the same movement as done by two different people.

The Daddy Series is for daddies, grandparents, babysitters, caregivers, friends, and other special people in your baby's life who might want to share yoga with your baby. The poses in the Daddy Series don't require any yoga experience, are easy to learn, and are very effective. If mommy isn't this book's main participant, then the Daddy Series can be shared with mommy.

Sleep Well Series

The Sleep Well Series can help transition your baby to sleep. It is best practiced during your baby's bedtime routine or when he awakens in the middle of the night. Dim the lights and soften any background noise or stimulation as much as possible. If your baby is accustomed to falling asleep with recorded music, play it ever so softly in the background or replace it with soft underlying white noise. Perhaps your baby falls asleep without any background sounds and that's fine. There is no need to add music now. Change your baby-yoga voice to a slow, soft but audible whispering voice and be sure to have a glass of water nearby to keep your throat and mouth moist. Your touch should communicate mindfulness, calm, and a sense that you will be with him as he sleeps. Let your strokes be longer, slower, mindful, and in a sense deeper so that the memory of your loving touch will last with your baby as he stays fast asleep. Change the velocity of each pose by allowing yourself more time to complete each one. Make the movement of the poses slower and more calming. All elements of your baby's yoga practice will communicate that it is time for bed, in every sense.

About the Practice of Series

It's best to practice the series within your baby's current developmental stage, but you can also go back and revisit series from previous stages. Each series includes poses from the chapter you are currently practicing as well as past poses. I strongly recommend that you do not move ahead in the book and put your baby into yoga poses that are designed for more physically mature and older babies. It is important for your baby to learn new poses that are appropriate for his development while maintaining a level of continuity and repetition that is healthy for him. Where you practice the series with your baby is up to you. No elaborate setup is needed for the yoga series to take place. Itsy Bitsy Yoga is about you and your baby. The rest of the world can wait.

Two Techniques of a Baby's Yoga Practice

Parents and babies usually come to yoga for one of two reasons, a Quick Fix or a Bond & Be Well practice. Itsy Bitsy Yoga is practical because I give you the tools for yoga to fit into your needs and schedule. After learning the fundamentals you can choose the Quick Fix or Bond & Be Well technique for your baby's yoga practice.

Quick Fix Technique

The Quick Fix Technique is exactly that, a quick fix. Use it to resolve an issue. Some babies have more issues than others, but all issues need tending to, and yoga can help you. During a quick fix situation, practice a Magic Pose, Happy Baby Series, or any posture your baby absolutely loves!

Quick Fixes typically happen on the go, without a blanket and soft music. It's just you remaining calm and making your baby happy! Quick fixes can easily take place outside the home. Moms and dads tell me stories of practicing Quick Fix techniques in the grocery store, at a relative's home, in parking lots, and on vacation.

Bond & Be Well Technique

The Bond & Be Well yoga practice happens when you follow any of the Itsy Bitsy Yoga series or the appropriate developmentally based yoga chapter for your baby. This book will teach you more than seventy yoga poses exclusively for your baby from birth to age two.

If I had my choice every baby would be happy *always*. Since that is not the case, we need to start where our babies are. When your baby isn't happy and content use the Quick Fix Technique. And when your baby is calm use the Bond & Be Well Technique.

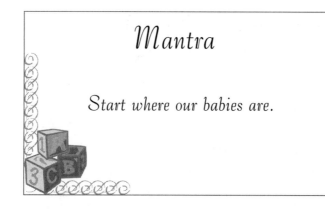

Mantra

Start where our babies are.

Quick Fix Technique

- No ambience
- Practiced anywhere
- Practiced whenever there is an issue
- Duration is 20 seconds to 5 minutes

Bond & Be Well Technique

- Ambience
- Generally practiced at home
- Practiced anytime
- Duration is 5 to 25 minutes

Twins

If you have twins, congratulations—you have twice the joy and benefits of a baby yoga practice. In teaching a number of twins, I find that it is best to practice a series with one baby and then the other. As your twins get older you can engage with one baby for a series of poses while one watches and then do the same series with your other baby. Take turns alternating who goes first. Begin to notice if your twins' favorite poses are the same or different. Also, if you have someone helping you, perhaps he or she can practice yoga with one baby as you work with the other.

Elements of the Developmentally
Based Yoga Chapters

Six of the seven developmentally based yoga chapters contains ten yoga poses and one contains eleven poses that can take around twenty minutes to complete. (Those who have become familiar with the poses may need less time; and others may wish to spend a little longer in relaxation.)

Do not rush on to the next developmental chapter. Stay with the ten or so developmentally appropriate poses for as long as your baby is in that stage. Your baby thrives on repetition. The more times she does something the better she becomes at it and the better she feels about it.

Now let's look at the unique components of Itsy Bitsy Yoga you will find within these chapters.

Meet Baby Spirita

 I am Baby Spirita. My job is to convey the benefits of each pose to you at the beginning. Helen tells me that I am the wisdom and voice of babies everywhere.

What Is a Mantra?

The word *mantra* is a Sanskrit word derived from "man" (mind) and "tra" (deliverance). Stated simply, a mantra is a sound vibration that resonates through your mind. One of my favorite Itsy Bitsy Yoga mantras is *Like spit, yoga happens.* Throughout the book you will find friendly little mantras to help keep things simple!

Introducing the Sing & Do Technique™

 I love to be talked and sung to. Imagine how horrible it would be if someone cared for you all day long but didn't speak to you directly. It would make you feel so lonely and unimportant. Remember, I love the tone of your familiar voice whether you're singing or talking.

Adults usually don't talk through yoga practice, but I believe yoga for babies and toddlers is quite different. The Sing & Do Technique is unique to Itsy Bitsy Yoga and I incorporate it into many of the postures I've adapted from traditional yoga or developed through my experience with babies and toddlers. As an example, here is a line from Hop Along Yogi's Sing & Do Technique:

♪ ♪ Sing & Do

Toes	Hold baby's left foot near her ankle.
To the	Bring baby's toes to the nose.
Nose	Tickle nose with toes.

Sing & Do is a musical inflection of the speaking voice to communicate respect, set the tempo of the movements, create a calm space, help babies and tots learn through repetition and predictability, and deepen the parent-child bond.

A parent's voice in the Sing & Do Technique is essentially that slow and melodic speaking voice that experts refer to as "parentese." Parentese is the kind of speech best suited to helping babies learn to talk. Please don't underestimate babies' grasp of what we are saying to them. They are conscious beings in little bodies. Well before they can respond with words or sign language, babies and toddlers can understand a lot of what is said. As a baby's yoga practice and mobility grow, the Sing & Do Technique engages and keeps a baby's attention on yoga and fun!

Six Reasons to Use the Sing & Do Technique

1. It develops the brain.
2. It communicates respect.
3. It sets the tempo of movements.
4. It is repetitive and predictable.
5. It awakens your inner child.
6. It reflects contentment.

Brain Development

Singing to your baby has a profound effect on his brain development. Researchers believe that singing engages more language centers in a baby's brain than do words alone. One sweet sixteen-month-old girl, Emma, learned to sing the words "I love you" by practicing the I Love You! Pose (page 95). A non-walking eighteen-month-old baby, David, learned how to sing his name before he could say it and would join us in Name Singing (page 101) during class.

Communicate Respect

Many times the words in Sing & Do are names of body parts or the posture's name. This helps a baby recognize the postures and become familiar with her own body parts or movements. A perfect example of this is Baby Planet (page 78). In fact, Serina's mom uses Baby Planet to help get Serina dressed in the morning. Your baby is an active participant in yoga practice, and by telling her about her movements you are respecting her. The times in between words and poses give your baby the opportunity to communicate back with you.

Tempo of Movements

The Sing & Do Technique sets the tempo of movements so that parents can learn the posture's pacing. Going too quickly is likely to overstimulate and upset the baby.

Repetition and Predictability

Babies thrive on repetition; it's how they learn. The repetitive and predictable patterns in Sing & Do let a baby predict what's next. For active babies and tots, the Sing & Do words actually prompt a baby to initiate or move into the pose. Remember Trevor, who went right into Tree Pose the moment he heard his mom utter those words.

Awaken Your Inner Child

At times, Sing & Do involves my spinoffs of classical nursery rhymes—for example, Ring Around the Yogi instead of Ring Around the Rosie. Movement-based songs bring tranquility into the room, comforting both parent and baby. Music is like a time machine, bringing parents back to a wonderful place in their own infancy. Sing & Do creates a harmonious feeling between you and your baby.

Reflect Contentment

Singing reflects a state of balance and a positive inner glow of contentment and equanimity. When we are emotionally upset, singing is very difficult, if not impossible. Babies are extremely sensitive to the way those around them feel. When you are calm, your baby is clam.

Ready to Start?

Regardless of when you begin this book, please read the Yoga Fundamentals chapter that precedes the developmental stage your baby presently occupies. Chapter 3, Infant Yoga Fundamentals, sets the stage for sharing yoga with a pre-crawling baby. Chapter 8, Tots Yoga Fundamentals, is for active crawlers up to twenty-four months old. Both chapters give guidance on developing a baby's yoga practice, and should be read before you and your child begin doing yoga poses. This is where you'll learn to prepare yourself and your environment for a successful yoga practice with your baby.

Through years of experience in developing my program I have placed the poses where they are best suited to a baby's current stage of development. As your baby grows so can his yoga practice, and you can revisit past chapters. So whatever age your baby is, please begin with the chapter best suited to your baby's developmental stage. Later you can go back and practice poses from any previous stages.

Anything Else I Should Know?

Keep in mind that yoga can be like other exercise or movement classes; there will be some exercises or poses you like more than others. Your baby will have the same sentiment. Each pose, each day, and each baby is different. If you have a sibling, think about how different the two of you are, even though you have the same parents. Each baby will have a slightly different experience of yoga. Your baby's experience will change as her body does. I respect all that appears and hope you do too!

How Often Should My Baby Practice Yoga?

Yoga can be practiced once or many times throughout the day. Commit to sharing yoga and your full attention with your baby, whether it be once a week or three times a day.

Chapter 3

Infant Yoga Fundamentals

Hi again! I'm Spirita and I do not crawl yet but I sure do love yoga! If your baby is not crawling either, this chapter will get you started in preparing your mind, your baby, and your environment for yoga and relaxation with your newborn, headholder, almost-sitting, or almost-crawling baby. Once your baby starts to crawl refer to Chapter 8, Tots Yoga Fundamentals. It provides an overview on how to successfully share yoga with your mobile baby.

This is a wonderful time to begin yoga, whether your baby is a newborn, a head-holder, almost sitting, or almost crawling baby. Itsy Bitsy Yoga is a gentle, loving practice that allows parents and babies get to know each other better. Infants practice yoga on their backs, bellies, or in your arms. Through observation and gentle facilitation you will guide your baby into positions and movements that will increase his comfort and joy as his body and mind develop!

Itsy Bitsy Yoga gives you additional tools and techniques for holding, moving, and calming your baby. In this chapter you will learn how to get started in sharing yoga with your infant.

Babies are extremely sensitive and are affected by how others feel. Have you ever been in a room with several babies and when one baby starts to cry the other babies begin to cry too? Babies are unaware of where they stop and where the world begins. To help you find a calmness within yourself I will teach you how to do Belly Breathing in this chapter. As parents breathe with the mindfulness of belly breathing they can better assist their babies in achieving a calm state. Through yoga, you and your baby's world merge and nothing else seems to matter—it's just you and your baby.

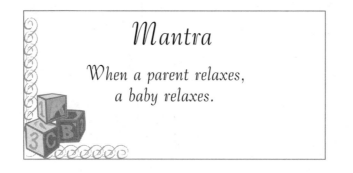

Mantra

*When a parent relaxes,
a baby relaxes.*

Set the Space

Set the ambience of your yoga space to include things that induce relaxation for you. Use natural or soft lighting. Add some soft music, perhaps the same music you played for your baby while you were pregnant. If possible, clear away any clutter. By eliminating things that distract you, you are eliminating the very things that pull you away from being with your baby during your special yoga time.

During most of your baby's yoga practice you will be seated. Practicing yoga on the floor covered with a rug, padded blanket, or yoga mat is ideal. However, if you find sitting on the floor difficult, adapt your practice and sit on a couch or bed. Keep your baby's safety and comfort a priority as you bring yoga off the floor and onto a bed or couch.

 As a young baby, I use my nose to search for my parent's natural body scent so we can bond or I can nurse. If the room becomes filled with incense or perfume it impedes my ability to smell my parent.

Props

You can temporarily transform a space in your home into a yoga space by including the following:

- **Pillows** help make you and your baby comfortable. Many people like to use a pillow under their head or knees during relaxation. If you are nursing your baby, try placing a pillow under your elbow as well as under your baby.
- **Calming music** can add another level of special ambience when practicing Itsy Bitsy Yoga. I tend to play soft instrumental music. Anything by Steven Halpern works well. Also try to play some of the music you may have shared with your baby during pregnancy.
- **A small toy or rattle** will help you guide your baby's head in turning toward a particular direction. A small toy can also engage a more active baby's upper body as you share yoga.
- **A receiving blanket** is your baby's yoga mat.
- **A mirror,** full length if possible. It is so much fun to practice poses in front of a mirror that allows you to see your baby's reactions when she is facing outward.

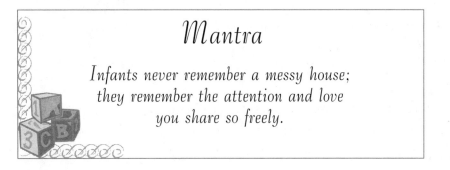

Mantra

Infants never remember a messy house;
they remember the attention and love
you share so freely.

Your baby will bond to what's near him just as you are bonding to what's near you. Remember, the way you're feeling is part of a baby's environment. You can share yoga with your infant in any room of your house. If you find that one location doesn't seem to be working out, try another.

Some babies are sensitive to certain locations within a room. I have often seen a baby's alarm go off. Once when I heeded my intuition and suggested that the parent and baby move to different part of the room, the baby's unexplainable crying stopped.

Set the Mood: Belly Breathing

A common breathing technique used in yoga is Belly Breathing. When practiced before yoga, Belly Breathing helps makes you more relaxed, calm, and confident.

How to Belly Breathe

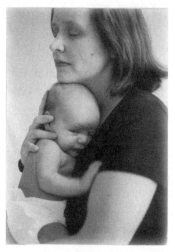

Sit comfortably with a tall, erect spine. Place your baby close to you. Perhaps she can lie across your lap or on her back with her legs near yours. Shrug your shoulders up and then roll them down and back. This will invite your chest to open (freeing the love and energy in your heart to shine and expand). Place your hands on your thighs with palms up. Bring your elbows in, close to your sides, and shoulders down. Breathe in and out through your nose, long, deep, and slow.

As you inhale, fill your tummy, like a balloon. Continue inhaling until you have completely expanded your chest as well. Now, "sip" in even more air! Feel those lungs stretch! Pause and hold it without "locking up." (If you are pregnant, do not hold your breath.) Gradually, increase the time you hold the inhale from a few seconds up to a minute as you progress in your practice.

Exhale completely. Empty yourself of breath by contracting your hips, then your abdominal region and finally your diaphragm. Let your heart feel like it is pressing toward your spine and down toward your belly button. Squeeze it all out!

Do this three to eleven times before each yoga practice.

 After my birth I practice my yoga or yogic breathing (or pranayam) naturally. After being born, I breathe only through my nose. I am never concerned with the past or future. I am always in the present moment. This awakened state I live in is what yoga and meditation practitioners strive to achieve.

Dressing for Yoga

Dress comfortably, avoiding any clothing that restricts movement for you or your baby. Whenever the room temperature allows, practice yoga with your baby in a diaper.

Set Your Intention

Your subconscious mind is like a computer; it does what you enter. For that reason, create a positive intention before practicing Itsy Bitsy Yoga. You can choose any of the intentions I've provided for you or write one of your own:

- Yoga is special for my baby and me.
- I am the perfect parent for my baby and my baby is perfect for me.
- I remain relaxed as I notice and fulfill my baby's needs.
- I trust my intuition.

Honor a Baby's Wishes

Now that your intention is set it is important that you honor your baby's intentions, too. Yoga is not something you do to your baby—it is something she does with you. In teaching adults yoga, I ask my students if I may place my hands on them to assist them in the postures before doing so. Similarly, request permission from your baby before helping her do yoga. Gauge the response to see if her body language indicates a yes or no. Babies respond to poses differently from day to day, especially earlier in life. A baby's response to yoga can change from moment to moment depending on her needs for food, comfort, cleanliness, or sleep. A baby's physical health and growth can also change her response to yoga poses.

A baby is born with his own will and desires. Adults should not feel as if their will can be imposed on a baby. If your baby becomes hungry or tired during yoga it is important for you to stop the practice and fulfill his wishes. It is your goal to identify and support your baby's needs, even when you wanted to try another pose or two. Itsy Bitsy Yoga teaches respect and opens the lines for clear communication later in a child's life.

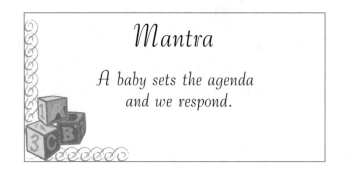

Mantra

*A baby sets the agenda
and we respond.*

Announcing Transitions

Let a baby know what happening and what's coming next by speaking to her. Let her feel that daily life isn't something that just happens but something that she is participating in and understands as it is happening. Softly announce transitions to your baby: for example, "I am going to pick you up now." Some parents like to even give babies a count to follow: "I am going to pick you up; one, two, three . . ." and by "four" the baby is in her parent's arms. Give babies enough time to register the activity at hand. Let the transition from holding her to your chest to placing her on a blanket be slow. Give a baby time to follow the activity in her body and mind.

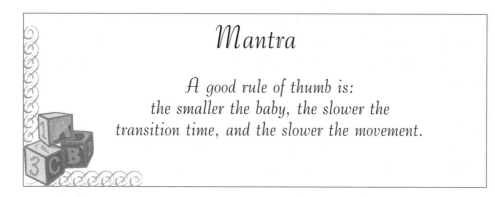

Mantra

A good rule of thumb is:
the smaller the baby, the slower the
transition time, and the slower the movement.

Reading Your Baby's Body Language

As you and your baby practice yoga you'll begin noticing your baby's movement preferences. Your baby's early preferences and body language may offer clues about how to approach activities with your baby. Below, I share some of these clues with you so that your baby's yoga practice is something that your baby has a say in!

If your baby becomes stiff . . .
   Use a lighter touch and resume the movement or pose at a slower, gentler pace.

If your baby is super flexible . . .
   Facilitate the pose as described and enjoy it. Don't worry about taking a baby deeper into the pose.

If your baby likes to watch first . . .

Use a doll, stuffed animal, or yourself to demonstrate the pose. This allows your baby to see the pose before experiencing it. This is particularly helpful with older babies and tots.

If your baby seems to look off to one side . . .

Stop facilitating the movement and leave your hands in place on your baby's body. Begin to sing to your baby until you make eye contact, and let him follow your eyes and head to center. Slowly resume. Many babies exhibit a side preference early in life. To balance visual sidedness, place interesting toys on the side that your baby favors least visually.

If your baby arches her back off the floor . . .

This is one way a baby communicates "No thank you." When a baby strongly arches her back, please respect the baby's cue of refusal by pausing to see what her needs are. Then you can determine if she is willing to move on to the next pose.

If your baby likes it active . . .

Follow the pose as described but increase the velocity of the swinging, rolling, and floating poses incrementally and safely. Practice with gusto and grace by letting the movements be large and full of life.

Reading Your Baby's Cries

If your baby is crying, breathe deeply and try to remain calm. No one hears your baby crying as loudly as you do. Use your intuition or a checklist (hungry tired, needs to be changed, wants affection, wants to move) to determine what the cry is trying to communicate. Always interrupt a baby's yoga practice to take care of needs such as changing a diaper, feeding, sleeping, or holding. When your baby is fed, alert, and freshly diapered it is a perfect time to practice a Magic Pose or another of your baby's favorite yoga poses.

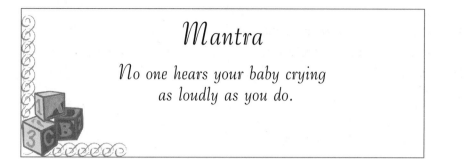

What happens if my baby gets fussy during a yoga pose?

1. Breathe!
2. Slow down the movement or pose.
3. See if your baby has an immediate need (for food, sleep, or an affectionate hold).
4. Stop and recheck the pose's directions.
5. Try it again in a week or two when your baby is slightly older.
6. Move onto a Magic Pose then resume with the next pose in the series or chapter.

As You Begin

Yoga can take anywhere from twenty seconds to twenty-five minutes. The reward is tremendous joy or bliss for you and your baby. Read the directions for each pose before sitting down to practice them with your baby. This will help focus your attention on the experience itself rather than on the words in the instruction. When you share a new yoga pose with your baby start with the minimum number of repetitions. Slowly increase the number of repetitions up toward the maximum as it suits your baby. With repeated practice you and your baby will become more experienced with the poses and your practice together will flow beautifully.

Experts and parents alike say a good baby is a predictable baby. Therefore, I believe babies feel good when their parents or caregivers are predictable. That's another reason to remain dedicated to fostering healthy routines into your baby's day, especially when you're busy.

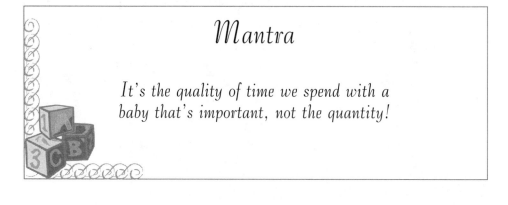

Mantra

It's the quality of time we spend with a baby that's important, not the quantity!

Positioning

As you practice the poses, I refer to a few common positions that serve as a starting position. Rather than repeatedly explaining a simple hold position I will refer to the Newborn Cradle, One-Handed Burp Hold, and Diaper Seat Hold. I will explain each to you here. If they are unfamiliar to you, practice them now.

Newborn Cradle
Used in Chapter 4, Yoga for Newborns
Wrap a towel or receiving blanket round and round into a long rope. Make it into a horseshoe shape (or upside-down U-shape). Let this rolled towel cradle your baby's head and body, thereby keeping her head straight.

One-Handed Burp Hold
Used in Chapter 4 and in Chapter 5, Yoga for Head-Holders
Bring one hand under your baby's chin, with your thumb near one of your baby's cheeks and your index finger near the other. Hold your baby as directed in the posture. This supportive hold helps younger babies keep their heads upright.

Diaper Seat Hold

Used in Chapters 4, 5, 6, and 7

While you are sitting or standing, place your baby's back against the center of your chest. From behind your baby, reach your right hand underneath your baby's diaper and spread your fingers as if you are giving her tush a seat to sit on. With your left hand use the One-Handed Burp Hold described above to maintain your baby's head upright.

 By placing me in the Diaper Seat Hold, I still feel supported by you but I can see the world in front of us. This position prepares us to do fun postures like Divine Drops and Swirlie that babies like me absolutely love!

Family Involvement

It can take a small village to raise a baby. Let others get involved in helping you with chores and errands so you can be with your baby, or let them practice yoga with the baby so you can take a shower or relaxing bath. The Daddy Series contains the perfect assortment of yoga poses that dad feels comfortable doing and are easy for him to follow—or for you to show him. Dads deserve and need to bond with their children. A dad's touch, presence, and love are extremely important to a baby and later child—and Mom values it too! Studies show dads who bond with their babies in the first weeks and months after birth have a deeper bond with their children throughout their lives.

A nice way to follow the poses in this book is to involve your spouse or a friend, babysitter, or other family member. Let them read the instructions to you one day while you share yoga with your baby and then, next time, switch.

Yoga is a great family activity. If your baby has older siblings, let them practice yoga with you and your baby. Children of all ages love to engage in movement and yoga poses. Olivia, a twenty-three-month-old who started yoga with me at ten weeks, now has a little brother, Justin. Olivia rubs her hands together and shares Heart-Warm Touch and Tiny Tugs with Justin. Siblings of all ages might like to share yoga with their new little sister or brother.

Humans beings grow in many ways: spiritually, physically, emotionally, and intellectually. The array of experiences you share with others ultimately deepens your own growth. Your baby is here to teach you and you are here to teach your baby. You bring life lessons to each other. Through yoga you are given an opportunity to witness and facilitate growth on all levels. Yoga can help you recognize growth as a gift.

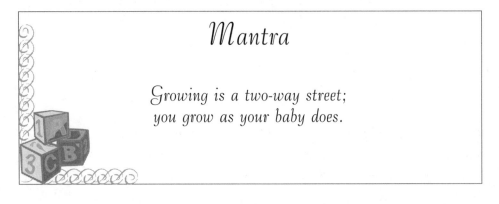

Mantra

*Growing is a two-way street;
you grow as your baby does.*

The Five B's of Itsy Bitsy Yoga

1. Be Love
Love is a calm and compassionate touchstone for a family.

2. Be Present
Presence means you are temporarily free from worry and hurriedness.

3. Be Listening
Listening is hearing what a baby's cries, smiles, and movements may mean.

4. Be Responsive
Responsiveness is giving your babies what they need.

5. Be Gentle
Gentleness facilitates your baby's experience of Itsy Bitsy Yoga.

When to Practice

It is best to practice yoga with a baby who is fed and not overly tired. If you know when your baby's witching hour is, try to practice five or more yoga poses about forty-five minutes prior to your baby's fussy time of day. You may notice a difference. Remember, your baby can enjoy a Bond & Be Well practice or a Quick Fix practice. Yoga can happen with your infant in the morning, afternoon, evening—or in the middle of the night. Your baby can practice as much yoga as she is willing to. There are so many poses and series to choose from! NOTE: Yoga should *not* be practiced while your baby is feeding or sleeping.

Yoga After a Feeding

Adults typically wait sixty or more minutes after eating before they practice yoga. Babies are different; they can practice most yoga postures shortly after eating. Babies are typically happy when full, and just like us they sometimes need to move in order to aid digestion. Think of how much a good walk can help you digest a meal. Gentler yoga poses, especially those in the Good Morning or Sleep Well series, are safe bets after a feeding. Trust your instincts and avoid any bouncy or rollie yoga poses with your baby for thirty minutes after your baby has eaten. This will lessen the chance of your baby spitting up.

Yoga and Reflux

If your baby has reflux, yoga is good for her. Building tone around her entire digestive tract is helpful in maturing your baby's digestive system. If your baby's reflux is severe, use an inclined position to elevate her head slightly higher than her stomach. For the yoga poses babies practice on their backs, keep your baby on an slight incline. The Newborn Cradle described on page 30 may work, or you can create an incline with your thighs positioned at an angle and your feet on the floor. For head-holders and almost-sitting babies, you can use an infant bouncer seat (without toys attached) or Boppy. With reflux, keep a baby's head slightly higher than her heart during yoga.

Yoga and Side Dominance

When you practice yoga with your baby, alternate the starting side for side-differentiating poses like Padahasta (page 96) or Twinkle (page 75). This is similar to teaching your child how to brush his teeth with his right and his left hand. You may notice that starting on a particular side may not be as comfortable for you as the other is. This will help strengthen the sides of your baby's body and mind equally. On odd-numbered days I start with the left side, and on even-numbered days I start with the right side.

Ending with Relaxation

Someday you will be thankful that you taught me how to relax at such an early age. I am already thankful for everything you do for me. The time we spend relaxing together helps us bond and understand each other even more. We can begin to sense each other in new ways during this peaceful state.

After sharing yoga with your baby it is time for you to relax—baby willing, that is. Traditionally, a relaxation pose—Shavasana—concludes every yoga practice, with five minutes allotted for every half hour of practice. However, if you have the opportunity to share more than five minutes of relaxation with your baby, then go ahead and do so! If your baby is not willing to relax, don't get frustrated. Simply hold your baby, close your eyes, and move, sing, or dance with your baby. Let your baby's love, beauty, and innocence fill you as you relax in this more active fashion.

Relaxation Positioning Options

Heart-to-Heart, Belly-to-Belly So You Can Rest Pose:
Ideal positioning for newborns, head-holders, and almost-sitting babies.
Lie on your back and place a pillow under your knees. Propping the knees relieves lower back tension. Babies can lie on their bellies on top of their parent's or caregiver's chest.

Right Next to Me Relaxation Pose:
Ideal positioning for newborns, head-holders, almost-sitting, and almost-crawling babies.
Lie on your back and place a pillow under your knees if you'd like. Place your baby so that she is lying comfortably next to you as you relax.

Baby Sits, You Relax Pose:
Ideal for the almost-sitting, almost-crawling babies, and beyond
Lie on your back, with a pillow under your head if you'd like. Position your baby in a sitting position between your upper thighs with your baby's back closest to your torso.

Ahh, Relaxation!

The following words are expressed in one Indian greeting, *Namaste*. Try repeating them aloud to your baby before closing your eyes (or softly gazing) and resting into relaxation. Give your baby a toy to engage with.

> *I honor the place in you*
> *in which the entire universe dwells.*
> *I honor the place in you*
> *which is of love, of truth, of light, and of peace.*
> *When you are in that place in you,*
> *and I am in that place in me, we are one.*
> *Namaste.*

Now the Five- to Thirty-Minute Relaxation for You and Your Baby

1. Position your baby on her back next to you on the blanket. If your baby prefers to see everything, sit her between your upper thighs, using them to hold her in a safe, supported sitting position. Sometimes it helps to offer your baby her favorite small toy or teething ring. If at any time during relaxation you need to stop and reposition your baby, please do so.

2. Lie down and relax—you deserve it! Rest your arms at a 20- to 40-degree angle away from your body with the palms facing up. Let your eyes close and relax.

3. Feel your body touching the blanket, the floor, and then the Earth. Know that Mother Earth is here to support you and all her children. If anything is weighing heavily on your chest, mentally pick it up and put it aside. Let your heart open and shine.

4. Begin to release each of your muscles section by section. Gently "convince" your muscles to release their grip on your bones in order for new breath or *prana* to restore tense areas with new vitality.

5. Now, allow your eyes to rest back into their sockets. Your jaw can release its grip and relax. Silently tell yourself, "My face will relax, my face is relaxed." Replace the word "face" with other body parts, in turn. Starting at the top, work your way down your body, relaxing your face, throat, chest, shoulders, arms, hands, belly, lower back, hips, thighs, knees, calves, ankles, feet, and toes. Take the time to relax completely.

6. If your baby begins to babble during this mutual relaxation time, hear the sweetness of her voice (even consider making an audio tape of your baby's emerging voice). Try to keep your eyes closed if you know your baby is safe. Feel your body connecting with your baby on all levels.

7. Aim to enjoy this relaxation for five minutes initially. Gradually increase your relaxation time to fifteen or even thirty minutes. If you believe you might lose track of time, set an alarm or kitchen timer to

signal the close of your relaxation. Anytime you spend in relaxation will boost your energy and leave you feeling refreshed!

Mantra

Let your baby be the first person or thing you see when you open your eyes.

Ten Tips for Practicing Yoga with a Baby

1. Set the mood of the room for relaxation.
2. Relax yourself.
3. Ask your baby's permission to practice yoga.
4. Create a flow of energy and movement between you and your baby.
5. Go slow.
6. Use the Sing & Do Technique.
7. Notice your baby's cues.
8. Take breaks when your baby is hungry or tired.
9. Practice regularly.
10. Use positive reinforcement.

·················

Chapter 4

Yoga for Newborns

Even though I sleep a lot, I feel that we are getting to know each other. I am so glad to be here in your arms. I know that you love me and I hope you know I love you too!

Congratulations on being chosen as a parent or caregiver. This extraordinary baby came to you for a very special reason that you'll spend a lifetime helping her discover. Your baby has faith in you. She wouldn't be here if she didn't. She trusts you today and will for a long time to come as you continue to grow together. As your child begins to discover her surroundings and who she is, you are there with her as a touchstone of her past and future.

Mantra

*My baby has faith in me
and I have faith in my baby*

About three weeks after Andrew was born, I met him and his wonderful mother, Kelly, in an Itsy Bitsy Yoga class. She was so grateful for the arrival of her second baby, yet deep down she doubted herself and her ability to be a good mother for him. Everyone in yoga class could see what a wonderful, capable mother she was and how much she loved her son, but Kelly felt disconnected from her ability to care for her son. When Andrew was only a day or two old he had undergone surgery to help his digestive system function. After class, Kelly told me that something I had said made a difference to her. I told her and every mother in the class, "You are the perfect parent for your child." She realized that if Andrew had been born to another family he might not have survived his early digestive difficulties. Through practicing yoga and relaxation with her newborn, Andrew's mom began to realize that she was indeed the best mom for Andrew.

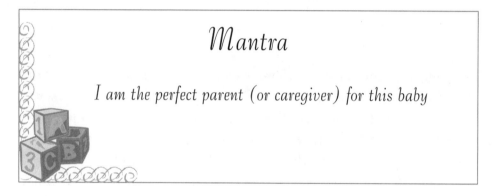

Mantra

I am the perfect parent (or caregiver) for this baby

Yoga can help increase your baby's ability to find a calm, comfortable state, ease in digestion, and a deeper bond with his new environment. In turn, this can make your transition to parenthood much more comfortable and satisfying. Your newborn is not too young to start benefiting greatly from yoga when practiced as described in this book. The three key areas we will focus on during Yoga for Newborns are:

- Calming
- Digestion
- Bonding

Calming is something most babies need assistance with, or have to learn how to do. Newborns often find calmness through touch or movement because it is familiar to them. In the womb, babies were held twenty-four hours a day and moved as much as their moms did. Techniques I share with you in this chapter to help bring forth calmness are Belly Breathing, Heart-Warm Touch, and Divine Drops.

Digestion is the act of assimilation, and sometimes we need to move to digest or assimilate what we have taken in. (Ever wonder why people go for walks after dinner?) In this chapter and throughout the book, I'll show you techniques and poses to help your baby digest effectively. In this chapter the poses particularly good for digestion are Chair Pose; Swirlies; One Hand, Two Hand; and Dolphin Pose.

Bonding is the awareness of the relationship between one's self and others. For parents and newborns bonding can take place through a shared steady gaze. As you hold and gaze at your baby, all the intelligence you need to become a wonderful parent is awakened. As your baby gazes back at you all the love, trust, and safety she needs for survival and growth is transmitted to her.

The gazes your baby gives to you will joyfully live in your heart for a lifetime. She treasures knowing that her beauty and the miracle of her being captivates your attention. Every time you gaze at your baby, you have the opportunity fall deeper in love with her presence in your life.

For bonding to take place, parent and baby should both be comfortable. So as you practice yoga, relax and be comfortable. This will make an ordinary yoga practice extraordinary. Belly Breathing, Setting Your Intention, the Heart-Warm Touch, Scoop n' Hug, and Bukka Bukka will strengthen the bond between you and your baby in this chapter.

The Present

Our babies are hardwired to exist in this moment. They are not concerned with what happened or can happen five minutes, five days, or weeks ago or from now. Because your baby is strictly concerned with the present moment, his concern in turn becomes your concern. Parenthood teaches you to listen so you can fulfill his needs for food, love, touch, movement, cleanliness, and sleep. Babies help us awaken our ability to center ourselves and be in this moment. As adults, we want to stick with our scheduled or current activity no matter how loud our babies' cries are. But as parents and caregivers we need to listen our baby's calls for something different.

Baby yoga helps you develop your flexibility in parenting. Flexibility means bending your needs and schedules around your babies' needs as they learn to find a schedule. For most new parents this takes getting used to. When practicing yoga, if a need arises for your baby, stop and fulfill it. Before all else, remember your baby is utterly concerned with being happy, fed, and cared for in the present moment.

The Five S's of a Newborn's Yoga Practice

1. Start with minimum repetitions
2. Small movements
3. Slow down
4. Surrender your expectations
5. Stop as needed

Start with the minimum number of repetitions when you introduce a new pose to your infant. Work with the minimum number until you can complete the series and then start adding more reps into the mix. However, when you share any of my Magic Poses you can do as many as it takes to settle your baby into a calm, happy state.

The smaller the body, the smaller the movement will be. In Itsy Bitsy Yoga we facilitate movement. We never force our babies into moving against their will.

Slow all movements way down. As adults we are highly experienced movers and do things quickly. But babies are inexperienced movers, so their limbs should be moved slowly. This will help avoid overstimulating your baby. If your baby could be happier in any given pose, try slowing the pace of movement down even more than before.

Surrender your expectations, because this is your baby's yoga practice, not yours. Let your baby set the tempo. I instruct my students to set a goal of practicing one posture a day with babies under three weeks old. When more than one posture is practiced in a particular sitting during your baby's first twenty-one days, consider it a bonus.

Stop your baby's yoga practice as needed for diaper changes, feedings, sleep, and the like. Please don't get discouraged if you need to interrupt your baby's practice for any reason. It will always be there for you to return to. Some days you'll practice the ten postures one right after the other, but other days you won't even get through three poses. You and your newborn are still settling into a schedule. So when your baby has the desire to sleep, eat, poop, you need to honor that and fit yoga in when you can.

As you begin the yoga practice for newborn babies:

- Gather a towel or receiving blanket to create a head cradle for your baby to rest on (see page 30).
- Practice on your baby's changing table, a bed, or on the carpet or a blanket.
- Use pillows and soft music to make yourself comfortable.
- Start with Belly Breathing (see pages 24–25).
- End with a relaxation technique (pages 34–37).

One day an Itsy Bitsy Yoga mom, Ellen, had mustered the courage to take her newborn son, Simon, and her teenaged mother's helper to the beach. While at the beach, Simon was a little fussy and his mom started doing Divine Drops with him. Ellen was not afraid to practice yoga anytime and anywhere she saw the opportunity to. The mother's helper blushed and swore she wouldn't start the squatting movement while holding the baby in Divine Drops. The teen didn't think that Divine Drops would work, but Ellen knew better and continued until Simon's fussiness disappeared. From then on, the very things that the young mother's helper said that she would never do, she started doing every time Simon fussed no matter where they were.

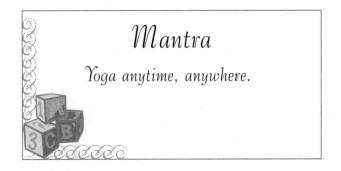

Mantra

Yoga anytime, anywhere.

Heart-Warm Touch

• • • • • • • • • • • • • • • • • • • •

(Newborn Version)

 I thrive on warm, loving touch. After gestating in the womb for months, nothing feels better than being skin-to-skin with you. Touch helps me to establish my ideal body weight as I feel the shell of this little body I now call home. Touch is also communicative and bonds me with my wonderful new family.

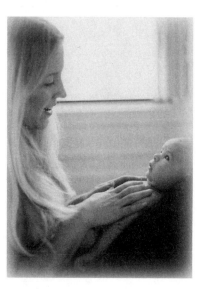

1. Sit comfortably on a cushioned surface with your back against pillows for support.

2. Prop your knees up 45 degrees directly in front of you, leaving your feet on the floor or bed.

3. Rest your baby on top of your thighs. He can face you with his feet closest to your belly.

4. Place the palms of your hands on your baby's tummy and chest. Take a few deep belly breaths (see pages 24–25).

5. Gaze softly at your baby, focusing on the rhythm of his breathing.

6. Close your eyes and imagine your heart and hands beginning to glow.

7. Begin to feel the warmth and love your baby is exchanging with you.

8. Place your left hand on his belly to keep him safely on your thighs.

9. Use your right hand to mindfully caress his entire body with a solid, predictable, loving touch.

 If I am having a monkey of a day, try just leaving your hands in place rather than caressing me. A deep, firm, predictable loving touch calms me.

10. Start at his shoulders and work your way down to the bottoms of his feet.

    NOTE: This is a slow stroke. A count of 6 "Yogaissippis" equals the time it can take for your hand to cover your baby's body length.

11. Continue for 30 seconds up to a minute as you bond with each other.

12. Exchange hands so your right hand supports him and your left hand caresses him. Repeat steps 10 and 11.

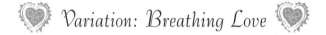

Variation: Breathing Love

Slowly lean forward so your head is near your baby's head. Let him see you or sense your presence. With soft lips and kindness softly blow your breath on your baby's head. Look for his reaction and repeat. Use this Breathing Love Technique whenever you want to share a calm smile with your baby.

Chair Pose
· · · · · · · · · · ·

Chair Pose helps me relieve any excess gas I may experience when learning how to digest.

1. Choose the position below that is comfortable for you.

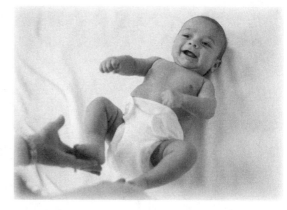

Start Position A:
From Heart-Warm Touch, lower your legs toward the floor while keeping your baby on top of your thighs.

Start Position B:
Rest your baby on her back and facing you on a blanket with another blanket or towel rolled up as a head cradle (see instructions on page 30).

2. Place the palms of your open hands on the bottom of your baby's feet.

Sing & Do

Chair   Push your palms away from you by a few inches. This flexes a baby's knees slightly toward her chest. Pause for approximately 6 to 10 seconds as you take a deep belly breath.

Pose   Bring the palms of your hands closer to you. This allows a a baby's legs to extend or lengthen.
Repeat 3 to 5 times.

3. Share the Heart-Warm Touch with your baby, gently extending her body.

Variation: Jiggle, Giggle Chair

Follow the directions above but instead of pausing with your baby's legs away from you, try jiggling her feet as if jiggling a piece of Jell-O up and down. This eliminates the pause and increases the tempo of step 2 to match an up-and-down jiggle motion.

Scoop n' Hug

· · · · · · · · · · · · · · ·

Scoop n' Hug is an opportunity for us to take time and do nothing but treasure each other. As you send me your loving positive feelings you are feeding my well-being. Even though it may seem as if I "take" all the time, I want you to be aware that I have love and appreciation for you too!

1. Continue to sit comfortably.

♪ ♪ Sing & Do

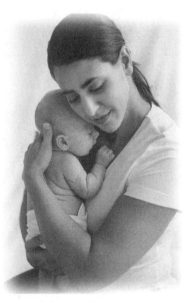

Scoop   Place your arms under your baby and slowly scoop him into an upright orientation.

n' Hug   Bring your baby to your chest and mindfully feel him close to you.

2. Use the One-Handed Burp Hold (see page 30) to support the back of his head. Your other hand can support his bottom as he remains resting at your chest.

3. In a moment, close your eyes and visualize your hearts connecting. Hear the beating of your hearts come together. Feel the strong bond that exists between the two of you.

4. Rest here for several minutes. There is no rush to move on to what's next. Just be here together.

Although my eyesight is still developing, my ability to hear your voice and feel your heartbeat is quite keen. During Scoop n' Hug our hearts beat together in a synchronized rhythm.

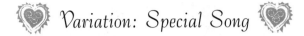 *Variation: Special Song*

When in Scoop n' Hug, softly sing your baby a song. Perhaps you have a song that uses your baby's name, or a special song that someone used to sing to you when you were little.

Bukka Bukka

• • • • • • • • • • • • •

(Bukka is the Sanskrit word for heart)

 Bukka Bukka recreates some of my favorite womb experiences. The light touch of your chin on my head feels like your uterine wall, and the closeness of our two hearts is familiar to me too! Thanks for making me feel at home as I enjoy the soft humming vibrations coming from your throat and chest.

1. Continue sitting comfortably and cuddle your baby's heart near yours.

2. Position your baby at the middle of your chest and vertical. She is facing you.

3. Lift your chin and nuzzle the top or crown of your baby's head under your chin.

4. Tenderly sing the words "I Love You," or gently say *Shhhhhhh*. Use a soft, resonating voice.

5. Continue for up to 45 seconds or for as long as your baby feels comfortable.

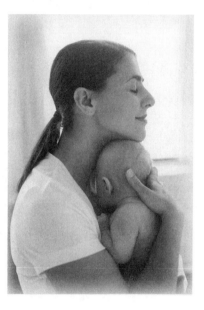

 Try practicing Bukka Bukka with me as you lie on your back. Having you under me helps me feel comfortable on my tummy!

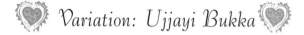

❤ Variation: Ujjayi Bukka ❤

Ujjayi (pronounced *oo-jai-eee*) breathing can calm both you and your baby. Follow the directions above but replace the singing of "I Love You" or *Shhhhh* in step 4 with Ujjayi breathing. Lightly close your lips and inhale the breath into your lower belly. Now imagine that you are about to fog up a mirror. Exhale just as you would to make the mirror fog, but keep your lips closed. As your breath sweeps across the soft palate of your throat you will hear an audible sound similar to an ocean wave. As you continue to inhale and exhale, let your jaw, tongue, and lips remain relaxed. Your inhale and exhale should be equal in length. Try starting with a 5-second inhale and a 5-second exhale and work your way up to 10 seconds. Use Ujjayi breathing while in Bukka Bukka with your baby or at any other time when you want to calm yourself and your baby.

Swirlies

· · · · · · · · ·

 By circling my hips clockwise you are tracing my intestinal highway and moving my poop through any traffic jams. In Swirlies I think of your hands as the start and finish line, with one hand on my stomach and the other under my diaper.

1. Sit with your legs in a V shape or stand comfortably with your feet more than hip distance apart.

2. Place your baby's back against the center of your chest in the Diaper Seat Hold as detailed on page 31.

3. With your right hand reaching under the center of his diaper, circle your baby's hips in a steady clockwise motion.

4. Keep his head supported and belly stationary with your left hand.

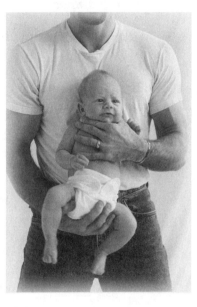

♪ ♪ Sing & Do

Swirlies   Slowly complete one clockwise circle of your baby's hip with your right hand.

5. Slowly repeat, circling your baby's lower body clockwise 3 to 5 times.

Divine Drops
• • • • • • • • • • • • •
(Newborn version)

Divine Drops activate my calming reflex and soothe me in a jiffy! Divine Drops are easy to do with me at anytime and almost anywhere—especially when I am in a fussy or colicky mood.

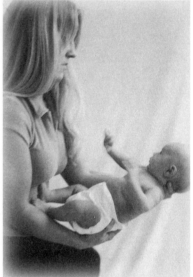

1. Stand with your feet more than hip distance apart.

2. Hold your baby facing you with her legs pressing into your abdomen. Place your right hand underneath her hips and lower back, and use your left hand to support your baby's neck and the back of her head. Her legs are being fully or partially supported as they snuggle into your body.

3. Turn your toes out to the sides in a 45-degree angle as you prepare to squat.

4. Inhale, filling your lower abdomen, chest, and arms completely with breath.

5. Exhale as you bend your knees and *quickly* drop down into a wide squat while continuing to hold your baby.

6. On your next inhale, press your feet into the floor and lift yourself and your baby back up into the starting stance.

♪ ♪ Sing & Do
Whhh   (inhale) Stand with feet more than hip distance apart.
Whoosh   (exhale) Quickly squat down while holding your baby.
              Repeat 3 to 10 times.

Magic Note: If using Divine Drops as a Magic Pose to calm your baby, it's important to match the intensity of her cries or fussiness with the speed of the drop and the number of repetitions.

For babies other than newborns, practice the Divine Drops Pose on page 79 with your baby facing outward.

I overheard Helen tell my parents that Divine Drops improves their digestion, increases flexibility in the lower body, and lengthens stiff back muscles. I am so happy this pose calms me and benefits my parents, too.

Note about Shaken Baby Syndrome and Yoga: Shaken baby syndrome is basically "baby whiplash." In Divine Drops and all other yoga postures described in this book you keep your baby's head in place, and supported.

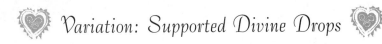

Variation: Supported Divine Drops

If you have back problems, a tired body, or if a baby becomes addicted to this pose, here are a few suggestions to make the pose easier. Try holding your baby as you bounce on a big plastic exercise or birthing ball. Or try holding your baby in a Diaper Seat Hold, place your back and hips against a smooth, empty wall, and position your feet about 12 to 18 inches in front of the wall. Keep your back and especially your shoulders against the wall during Divine Drops as you slide up and down the wall like an elevator.

One Hand, Two Hand

 One Hand, Two Hand brings awareness to the portion of my digestive tract where the stomach and small intestines meet. This is especially useful for me or any baby with reflux. The more that you help me experience touch and movement in this area, the easier it becomes for my body to keep breast milk or formula down.

1. Sit comfortably. Place your baby on his back with his feet nearest you.

2. Wiggle your thumbs into your baby's palms. Let your forefingers rest on top of his hands and wrists.

3. Using your baby's arms, gently cover and uncover his chest as you sing the One Hand, Two Hand song.

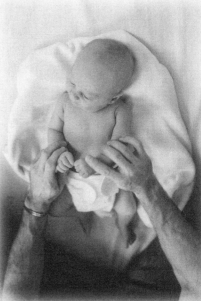

♪ ♪ Sing & Do

One Hand	Bring your baby's hands to his chest.
Two Hand	Caress and lower your baby's hands down his chest and out to the sides.
Three Hand	Bring your baby's hands to his chest.
Four!	Caress and lower your baby's hands down his chest and out to the sides.
I Love	Bring your baby's hands to his chest.
You	Caress and lower your baby's hands down his chest and out to the sides.
Forever	Bring your baby's hands to his chest.
n' More!	Gently wiggle his body from side to side, with his hands staying at his chest.
	Repeat once.

4. Applaud by clapping your baby's hands together and cheer "Yeahh!"

5. Finish with Heart-Warm Touch.

Tiny Tugs

 Tiny Tugs help me reach outward and discover the farthest points from my body's center. Tiny Tugs are extremely relaxing for you and me too!

1. In Tiny Tugs, we introduce a diagonal stretch to your baby by holding the opposite hand and foot and lengthening them away from each other.
2. Sit comfortably.
3. Slide your baby's hips close to you as she lies on her back in front of you.
4. Use your left hand to grasp your baby's nearest (right) hand with your thumb and first two fingers.
5. With your right hand, place your thumb on top of your baby's left foot (closest to your right hand). Your fingertips can rest around the bottom of her foot.
6. Lovingly give your baby's hand and opposite foot a gentle stretch.

Sing & Do

Tiny	Diagonally stretch hand and foot.
Tugs	Release the gentle stretch.
	Repeat 3 to 5 times.

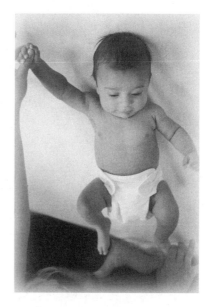

7. Switch sides and repeat step 6.
8. Share your Heart-Warm Touch with your baby.

Here & Now

Here & Now is a touch-stretch release technique that brings me to a place where my way of being and life's journey can unfold as they're meant to. As you continue yoga with me, our journey in life will become clearer to us both.

1. Sit comfortably with your baby resting on his back in front of you on his nesting cradle and facing you.

2. Use your left hand to hold your baby's right hand. Place your thumb in his palm and your first two fingers on top of his hand.

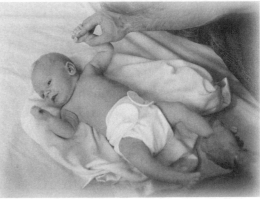

3. With your right hand, grasp your baby's right foot. Place your thumb on the bottom of his foot and your first two fingers on top of his foot.

4. Softly stretch and lengthen his arm and leg for 1 to 3 seconds.

Sing & Do

Here	Hold baby's right foot and hand.
and	Gently stretch and lengthen his hand and foot.
Now	Slowly release.
	Repeat 1 to 3 times, then switch sides.

5. Scoop your baby up and give him a nice hug!

Dolphin

 Dolphin Pose helps calm me. The tapping that you do at the base of my spine soothes my nervous system into a rhythmic, peaceful state. Most of the time it feels good to rest my belly on your thigh and look around! I sometimes think that Dolphin Pose is like a burp releasing whatever stress my body might have.

1. Sit with your back against a wall or similar surface. Prop your right knee into a 45-degree angle while keeping your foot on the floor.

2. Position your baby on her tummy along the front surface of your right thigh.

3. Slide your left hand between your thigh and your baby, and support her head in a burp-hold (thumb near one cheek and forefingers near the other). Most of your baby's body will be resting on your right thigh.

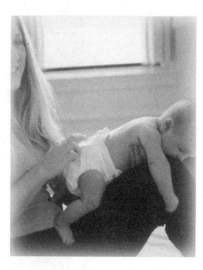

4. Locate your baby's sacrum by imagining that she is wearing tiny jeans. Her sacrum is where the middle belt loop on the back of her jeans would be.

5. Keeping the location of your baby's sacrum in mind, bring the first two fingers of your right hand together.

6. Use the tips of your first two fingers to gently tap on your baby's sacrum.

7. Continue tapping slowly and rhythmically for 5 to 30 seconds.

Experience the soothing sensation Dolphin brings to your nervous system by locating your own sacrum and tapping this point on yourself. If someone else is around, ask if they will tap for you so that you can enjoy the effect while they do the work for you!

Good Morning Series

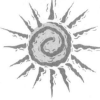

Yoga for Newborns

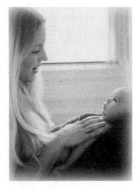

Heart-Warm Touch
page 45

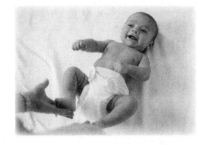

Chair Pose
page 47

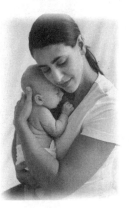

Scoop n' Hug
page 49

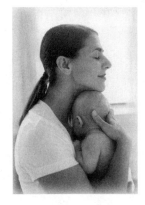

Bukka Bukka
page 51

Developmental Play Series

Yoga for Newborns

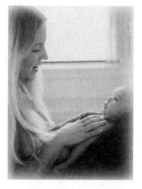

Heart-Warm Touch
page 70

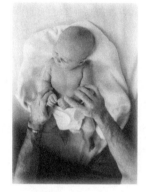

One Hand, Two Hand
page 56

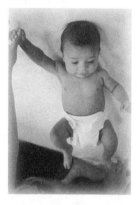

Tiny Tugs
page 57

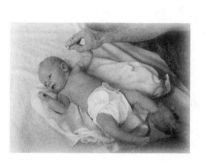

Here & Now
page 58

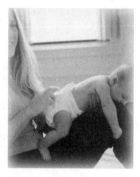

Dolphin
page 59

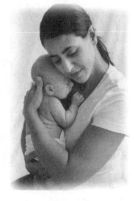

Scoop n' Hug
page 49

Happy Baby Series

Yoga for Newborns

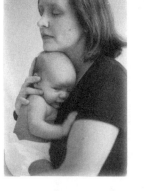

Belly Breathing
page 24

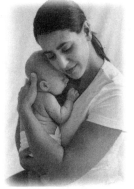

Scoop n' Hug
page 49

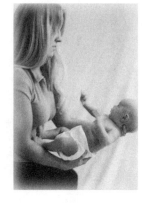

Divine Drops
page 54

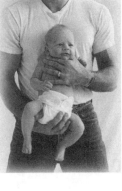

Swirlies
page 53

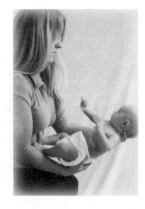

Divine Drops
page 54

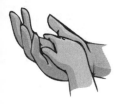

Daddy Series

•••••••••••••••

Yoga for Newborns

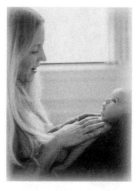

Heart-Warm Touch
page 45

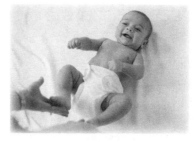

Chair Pose
page 47

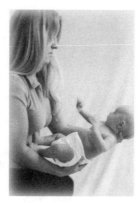

Divine Drops
page 54

Sleep Well Series

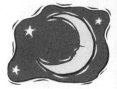

Yoga for Newborns

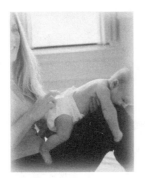

Dolphin
page 59

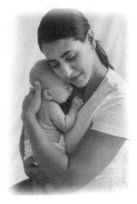

Scoop n' Hug
page 49

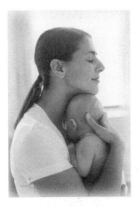

Bukka Bukka
page 51

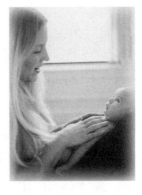

Heart-Warm Touch
page 45

Chapter 5

Yoga for Head-Holders

When you hold me upright close to you and my head doesn't fall forward, backward, or sideways, I'm ready to start the yoga poses for head-holders. I am also ready when I lie on my tummy with my head up and support myself on my forearms and tummy as I look around.

Do you notice your baby becoming more awake, alert, and interested in new ways to play and engage with you? Your growing baby is captivated with you and the external world. As a baby starts to support her head upright, her eyesight improves while her hearing remains keen. Right now, your head-holder is focused on lengthening the spine, toning the organs, and building muscle tone in the upper body. Perhaps one day soon you will find your baby's palms pressed onto the floor and her upper body lifted up as if she's in yoga's Cobra Pose.

Full-term babies are born before their bodies are fully ready to function efficiently; and major growth spurts are in store for babies within the first months after birth. An infant's birth weight may double before he can sit independently. Yoga can bring comfort to a baby's rapidly changing body. In Tibetan folklore, two invisible animals—the pig and the monkey—share in the caretaking of babies. When the pig tends to the baby, his flesh grows and the baby is quieter and sleeps better. On the monkey's day, the baby's bones grow, leading him to cry more with discomfort, and the baby does not sleep as well. When you focus solely on your baby during yoga practice, you are able to notice new developments and bodily changes.

As a baby matures and changes so do her likes and dislikes. What was uncomfortable three weeks ago may be very comfortable today. If you attempt a pose that your baby does not enjoy initially, try it again later. Remember, the baby's needs might taint her reaction to a pose. I have seen the re-exploration of yoga poses bring about deeply satisfying and positive changes in babies' reactions. As a baby grows, so will her repertoire of favorite yoga poses.

Using Yoga for Fussiness and/or Colic

Colic is a term used when a baby cries for at least three hours a day, three times per week, for three weeks. Luckily, colic is temporary and will pass. Colic tends to peak around six weeks after a baby's due date and fades away at about three months. Yoga can become a preventive measure for colic. If you have a fussy or colicky baby, the best time to share yoga with her is approximately forty-five minutes before your baby's fussiest time of day begins. When your baby is colicky or fussy it is not because you've done anything wrong. Remember, you are the perfect parent for your baby.

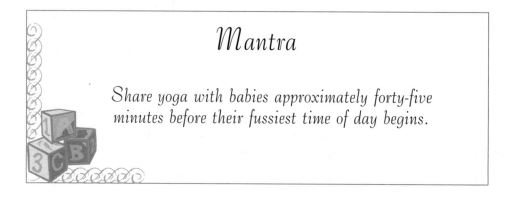

Mantra

Share yoga with babies approximately forty-five minutes before their fussiest time of day begins.

At eight weeks old, Alexander went to the doctor's office for several shots. Babies survive their shots, but how they'll react afterward is always questionable. Alexander's mom, Sarah, gave him a little Tylenol to soothe any pain and they went into the city to meet with friends. After about four hours, Alexander grew unusually irritable and fussy. Sarah and Alexander said goodbye to their friends and began their thirty-five-minute highway drive home. During this time, Alexander's irritability intensified into full-blown screaming and ballistic, unstoppable crying. Sarah was frazzled and tried to calm herself with deep belly breaths. She exited the highway and drove into an office-building parking lot. Sarah took Alexander out of his car seat and tried to calm him with a pacifier, with nursing, and by singing to him. Nothing was working. Then she recalled one of the poses she learned in yoga class, and she had a hunch it could ease Alexander's distress. Holding her screaming infant, Sarah squatted and rose through several Divine Drops (page 54). After eight to ten Divine Drops Alexander's crying fit lessened. Within fifteen Divine Drops he stopped crying completely. Sarah agrees Divine Drops is a Magic Pose. She is thankful for starting yoga with Alexander when he was four weeks old. Sarah had grown more confident and trustful of her parenting ability because of yoga.

Bonding Through Breath

Remember to take a deep breath when your baby is fussy. In the following activity we will explore bonding through breath. As babies begin to hold their heads up and lengthen their spines, they become more adept at Belly Breathing, which you learned on pages 24–25. Shared Belly Breathing can help bridge parent and child together.

1. Recognize How Your Baby Is Breathing

Begin to notice how your baby breathes through her nose exclusively. Observe the length of your baby's breath. Watch the movement of her body as she inhales and exhales. Newborns take about forty to forty-four breaths per minute compared to the average adult rate of twelve per minute. Notice how rapid your baby's respiratory rate is compared to yours.

2. Match Your Baby's Breathing Pattern

What can you notice about your breath? Are you breathing through your nose, mouth, or a combination of both? Begin to mimic and match your baby's breathing pattern, even if it seems a little awkward. Notice how you feel as you shift your breathing pattern to meet your baby's. Once you settle into your baby's breath pattern, how do you feel?

3. Find Breath and Comfort Together

As you and your baby bond through breath, find a level of comfort that suits you both. When we smile or belly laugh our breath naturally deepens, and our body relaxes as it fills with endorphins. Anxiety, crying, or screaming cause breathing to become shallow and the body to contract. Every sound a baby makes strengthens her diaphragm and increases her communication repertoire.

When I meet Laurie she was at her wits' end. Her baby, Samuel, wasn't sleeping for more than three-hour increments and he was often fussy or crying. Her friends had told her things would get better once her baby turned three months, but two weeks later things hadn't improved. Laurie was exhausted and ready to learn how yoga could help her family. The poses I used to help Laurie and her son are described in this chapter and focus on calming cries, improving sleep, and overall well-being.

Mantra

Yoga before bed for a good night's sleep!

As you begin practicing yoga for head-holders, you'll notice mature variations of two poses from Chapter 4, Yoga for Newborns: the Heart-Warm Touch and Divine Drops. The level 2 versions are suitable for your baby now, and throughout the rest of the book. Womb Wings and Baby Planet are well-loved by babies well into toddlerhood, so remember to revisit past poses as your baby's Itsy Bitsy Yoga practice blossoms.

As you begin the yoga practice for head-holding babies:

- Practice on your baby's changing table, a bed, or on the carpet or a blanket.
- Lay a receiving blanket out in front of you.
- Find a full-length or decent-sized mirror to practice yoga near.
- Play soft music.
- Start with Belly Breathing (pages 24–25).
- End with a relaxation technique (pages 34–37).

Heart-Warm Touch
· · · · · · · · · · · · · · · · · · ·

 Now that I am a little older I can rest on a blanket as you treat me to the Heart-Warm Touch with two hands at once. After practicing Heart-Warm Touch several times, I begin to know that it's time for yoga and relaxing with you. It feels so good to have your loving hands on me. Thank you.

1. Place your baby on a blanket, lying on his back with his feet nearest to you.

2. Relax using Belly Breathing (pages 24–25).

3. Rub the palms of your hands together above your baby to generate warmth and love.

4. Feel your heart beginning to glow with your favorite color. Imagine colorful and limitless loving energy pouring out from your heart and into your hands.

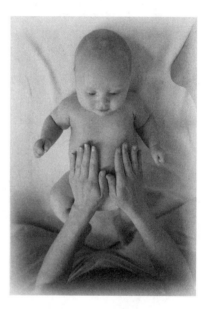

5. Bring both of your hands slowly to your baby's shoulders.

6. Starting at your baby's shoulders, move your steady Heart-Warm Touch all the way down his body to the tips of his toes.

NOTE: THIS A SLOW STROKE. A COUNT OF SIX (6) "YOGAISSIPPIS" MEASURES THE TIME IT TAKES TO SLIDE YOUR HANDS DOWN YOUR BABY'S BODY WITHOUT LIFTING THEM.

7. For up to one minute continue caressing the front and sides of his little body with this firm and predictable Heart-Warm Touch.

ABOUT COUNTER-POSES: LIKE TRADITIONAL YOGA, ITSY BITSY YOGA HAS COUNTER-POSES, OR THE POSE IN BETWEEN THE

POSES TOO. BEGIN TO SHARE AN ABBREVIATED VERSION OF HEART-WARM TOUCH AS A COUNTER POSE BECAUSE IT PLEASES BABIES SO.

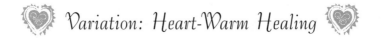

Variation: Heart-Warm Healing

Let your intuition guide you to a place on your baby's body that may need your loving, tender touch. Apply your heart-warm hands directly to that particular area. Leave your hands still for up to one minute. Try using Heart-Warm Touch on any scrapes or bumps that your little ones may endure. It is sure to comfort both you and your child!

A Magic Pose

Apana

● ● ● ● ● ● ●

(Apana is the Sanskrit word for waste)

 Mom or Dad, practice Apana Pose with me as often as we need to because it helps rid me of gas and constipation. You may notice that I seem to naturally bring my knees up toward my chest when digesting. I am grateful for your assistance as I learn about my body and how it works.

1. As in Heart-Warm Touch, your baby is lying on her back on a blanket with her feet closest to you.

2. Slide your thumbs between the blanket and the undersides of your baby's uppermost thighs.

3. Let your fingers rest loosely on top of her thighs.

4. Slowly lift your baby's knees up toward her chest.

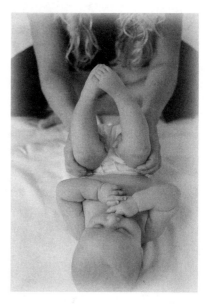

 Allow the degree of lifting to suit my wishes. If you begin to feel me resist, honor me and do not force my body's movement.

5. Hold your baby's knees in toward her chest for 3 to 10 seconds. This will aid your baby's digestion tremendously.

6. Slowly lower your baby's thighs toward the blanket.

7. Keep your hands cupped around your baby's thighs as they extend.

8. Repeat 3 to 10 times using the Sing & Do Technique.

Sing & Do

In	Lift baby's knees toward the chest.
and	Pause and hold knees toward the chest.
Out	Lower and extend baby's legs.

9. Don't forget to finish with the Heart-Warm Touch!

Variation: Less May Be More

If your head-holding baby is less than eight weeks old, the perfect Apana Pose may be a simple lift of the hips, without bringing the knees far up and into the chest.

Corkscrew

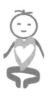

The long tunnel used in digestion is shaped like an upside-down triangle and flows in a clockwise direction. When my hips are circled clockwise in Corkscrew, we're following the natural route of digestion, helping make elimination a little easier in my new little body.

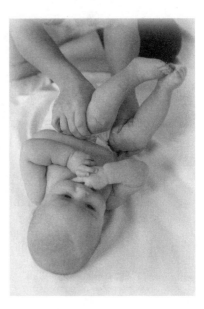

1. Let your baby rest on his back with your thumbs holding the back of his thighs and forefingers resting on top as in our last pose, Apana.

2. Begin to circle your baby's thighs clockwise with both hands.

♪ ♪ Sing & Do

Corkscrew Circle your baby's thighs, letting one circle equal the time that it takes to sing "Corkscrew."

3. Continue with Corkscrew for 5 to 30 seconds, keeping your voice and movement fluid and rhythmic.

Twinkle

· · · · · · · · ·

I love how you are so good at showing me how I can move through this world peacefully. In Twinkle, you are facilitating my arms so that I can start life without shoulder tension or tightness.

1. Place your baby on her back and slide her feet closer to you.

2. Entice your baby's palms to grasp your thumbs. Hold the tops of her hands with the first two fingers of each hand.

3. Use your left hand to lift your baby's hand into a soft 90-degree angle. (It looks as if your baby is raising her hand to ask a question in a schoolroom.) This is the *up* arm movement.

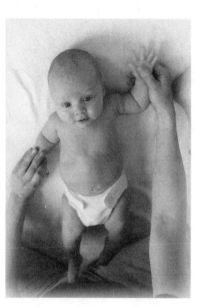

4. To practice the *down* arm movement, use the same hand to bring your baby's hand down by her side and waist.

5. OK, it's showtime!

 Sing & Do

Using your LEFT hand and baby's nearest arm:

Twin-	Up
kle	Down
twin-	Up
kle	Down
You're	Up
so	Down
bright	Rest

Using your RIGHT hand and baby's nearest arm:

Yo-	Up
ga	Down
helps	Up
you	Down
sleep	Up
at	Down
night	Rest

Using your LEFT hand and baby's nearest arm:

Up	Up
a-	Down
bove	Up
my	Down
heart	Up
so	Down
high	Rest

Using your RIGHT hand and baby's nearest arm:

My	Up
love	Down
for	Up
you	Down
fills	Up
the	Down
sky	Rest

6. That was great! Go ahead and share some positive words or affection with your baby.

Brain Builders

Brain Builders integrates the right and left sides of my body, including the right and left hemispheres of my brain. Brain Builders is a great way to maximize the possibility of future learning!

1. Baby is resting comfortably on his back with his feet closest to you.

2. With your left hand, hold your baby's right wrist by placing your thumb in his palm and your first two fingers on top of his hand.

3. Use your right hand to hold your baby's left thigh, diagonally opposite.

4. Simultaneously bring your baby's opposite hand and knee inward so that they meet or come close to meeting near his belly button while his shoulders stay on the floor.

If you are still telling people my age in weeks, my hand and knee may not meet together in Brain Builders. I really like how you honor my flexibility and remember that you are facilitating, not forcing my movements.

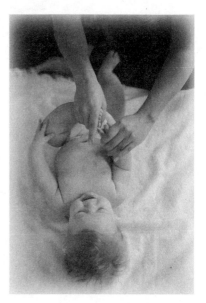

5. Let this Sing & Do have a nice long *shh* sound as you sing "Splish" or "Splash."

♪ ♪ Sing & Do

SpliSH	Bring your baby's hand and knee together.
SplaSH	Baby's hand and knee come apart.

6. Repeat 3 to 5 times before switching sides.

7. Treat your baby to your Heart-Warm Touch.

Baby Planet

Baby Planet teaches me navigational locations by bringing it all to a place where I learn best, in my body. Together yoga and the Baby Planet song help foster an awareness of space that helps me move with more confidence, grace, and skill.

1. Rest your baby on her back in front of you with her feet close to you.

2. Using both of your hands, follow the directions as you Sing & Do the Baby Planet song with your baby!

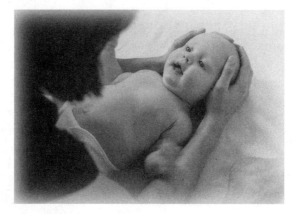

♪ ♪ Sing & Do

North Pole	Lightly touch your baby's head.
South Pole	Touch your baby's feet.
	Guide baby's hands to her chest if not already there.
East Coast	Open baby's left arm out to the side.
West	Open baby's right arm out to the side.
Inside	Bring in baby's hands to heart space.
Outside	Open both of baby's hands out to the side.
Baby, you're the best!	Wiggle your baby gently side to side.
	Repeat once or twice more.

Divine Drops

• • • • • • • • • • • • •

(Level 2)

In this version of Divine Drops I am held differently and get to face outward. This pose has calmed countless numbers of my baby friends in Helen's yoga class. Parents say they like to practice Divine Drops just about anywhere because it can make us babies giggle even when we're not in the mood to.

1. Begin by standing and holding your baby in a Diaper Seat Hold against your chest (see page 31).

2. Bring your feet about 18 to 24 inches apart so it looks like you are going into a squat.

3. Turn your toes out to the sides at 45-degree angles and continue holding your baby comfortably to your chest in the Diaper Seat Hold.

4. Inhale deeply, filling your upper body and torso with breath.

5. Exhale and bend your knees, quickly dropping down into a wide squat while continuing to hold your baby in place.

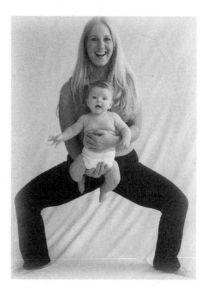

7. On your next inhalation, press your feet into the floor and rise back into the starting stance.

♪ ♪ Sing & Do

Mmm	Stand with feet 18 to 24 inches apart and toes out and inhale.
Whoosh	Exhale and quickly squat down while holding your baby in a Diaper Seat Hold.
	Repeat a minimum of 3 to 6 times.

If you have back problems, a tired body, or if a baby becomes addicted to this pose here are a few suggestions to make the pose easier. Try practicing Divine Drops on a big plastic exercise or birthing ball. Or hold your baby in a Diaper Seat Hold, place your back and hips against a smooth, empty wall and position your feet about 12 to 18 inches in front of the wall. Keep your back and especially your shoulders against the wall as you slide up and down the wall like an elevator.

 MAGIC NOTE: IF USING DIVINE DROPS AS A MAGIC POSE TO CALM YOUR BABY, IT'S IMPORTANT TO MATCH THE INTENSITY OF HER CRIES OR FUSSINESS WITH THE SPEED OF THE DROP AND THE NUMBER OF REPETITIONS.

Womb Wings

· · · · · · · · · · · · ·

Womb Wings lets my body move the same way that I floated in my mommy's womb. What a wonderful and familiar feeling that is for me!

1. Hold your baby in a Diaper Seat Hold as described on page 31.

2. Stand with your feet evenly spaced more than hip distance apart.

3. While holding her against your chest in a Diaper Seat Hold, bend forward from the waist without bending your knees.

4. Bend forward until you're close to being in a 90-degree angle or inverted L shape with the floor. For your comfort, keep a flat back.

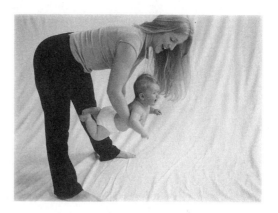

5. Reposition your hands so that one hand is under your baby's chest and the other under her legs.

6. Extend your arms while holding your baby away from you.

7. Your baby's chest and legs are several inches above the floor. Notice her limbs as they float freely.

8. Begin to rock your baby back and forth. Look straight ahead, keeping your spine long.

9. To keep a happy, playful tempo for your baby, sing the Womb Wings song as you swing your baby back and forth.

♪ ♪ ♪ Sing & Do

Womb	Forward
Wings,	Back
Womb	Forward
Wings,	Back
Womb	Forward
Wings,	Back
Woo!	Far forward
Womb	Forward
Wings,	Back
Womb	Forward
Wings,	Back
I love	Far forward
You!	Scoop her up into your arms and stand up.
	Repeat 1 to 3 times.

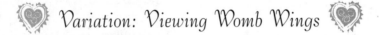

Variation: Viewing Womb Wings

If possible, try Womb Wings in front of a mirror to see if your baby is smiling. If she isn't smiling, but is fed and not tired, try Womb Wings again, going a little higher and faster.

One Foot, Two Foot Lotus

 One Foot, Two Foot Lotus is playful for me and incorporates something that big kids do—count with numbers. The position of my feet massages my belly and helps me become aware of my ankles, knees, and spine. That will later help me crawl, walk, and run.

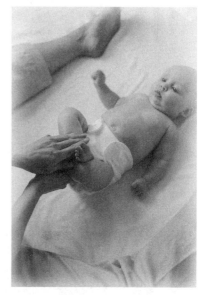

1. Sit comfortably with your baby lying on his back and facing you.

2. Place your thumbs just above each of your baby's outer ankles. Use your first two fingers to gently hold above the inner ankle area.

3. With your left arm, cross his right leg over his belly button and hold.

4. With your right arm bring your baby's left leg underneath his right leg. Hold for a moment.

5. Slowly uncross his legs.

6. Switch the bottom and top legs, so that baby's left leg is over his belly button with his right leg underneath.

7. Continue alternating your baby's legs into Lotus posititon as you sing the words to One Foot, Two Foot Lotus! (The words in the song are similar to One Hand, Two Hand; see page 56).

♪ ♪ Sing & Do

One foot,	Bring baby's LEFT leg across ABOVE his belly button.
Two foot,	Bring baby's RIGHT leg across BELOW his belly button.
Three foot,	Extend baby's LEFT leg LONG toward you.
Four!	Extend baby's RIGHT leg LONG toward you.
I love	Bring baby's RIGHT leg across BELOW his belly button.
You	Bring baby's LEFT leg across ABOVE his belly button.

Forever n'	Extend baby's RIGHT leg LONG toward you.
More!	Extend baby's LEFT leg LONG toward you.
	Clap the soles or bottoms of your baby's feet together!
	Repeat once.

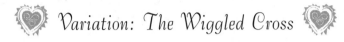 *Variation: The Wiggled Cross*

Each time you bring your baby's legs across his belly, give them a little wiggle.

Super Baby

One of the many reasons I love practicing the Super Baby Pose is that I have a rare bird's-eye view of you. With Super Baby, I get a new awareness of my body space, and it is a nice way for me to have my tummy time with you.

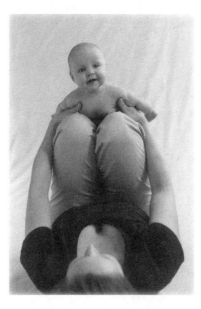

1. Bring your baby into your arms. If she has eaten within the past 30 minutes, you may want to practice the next pose or Shavasana Relaxation pose. You can come back to Super Baby when she is less likely to spit up.

2. Lie down with your baby on your belly.

3. Prop your knees into a 90-degree angle. Bring your knees and feet close together.

4. Place her belly side down on your shins so that your baby is looking down at you.

5. Leave your hands around her chest and waist to keep her safely in place.

Sing & Do

Super Baby Begin to bounce your baby on your knees.
Super Baby Roll your body and baby side to side (a nice lower back massage for you).
Super Baby Let your baby's reactions guide your movements.

6. Come out of Super Baby by lifting your baby and body into sitting. Give your baby a big hug! That was wonderful!

Variation: Super Name!

In Super Baby's Sing & Do Technique, replace the word "baby" with your baby's name. So perhaps it's "Super Annie!" or "Super Anthony!" By the way, your baby will start responding to her name soon if she hasn't already.

Good Morning Series

· ·

Yoga for Head-Holders

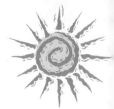

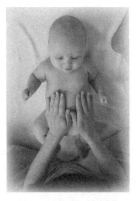

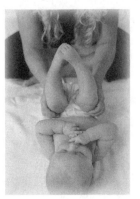

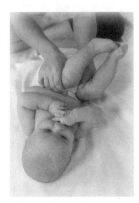

Heart-Warm Touch
page 70

Apana
page 72

Corkscrew
page 74

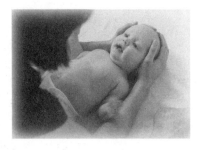

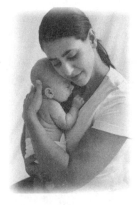

Baby Planet
page 78

Scoop n' Hug
page 49

Developmental Play Series

Yoga for Head-Holders

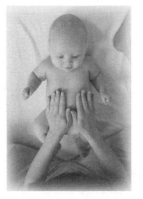

Heart-Warm Touch
page 70

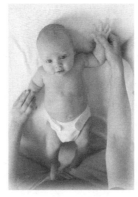

Twinkle
page 75

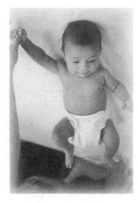

Tiny Tugs
page 57

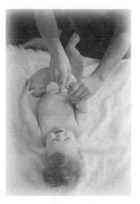

Brain Builders
page 77

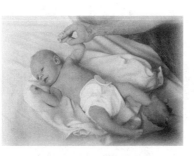

Here & Now
page 58

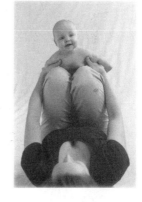

Super Baby
page 85

Happy Baby Series

Yoga for Head-Holders

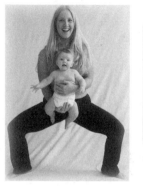 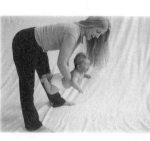 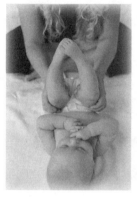 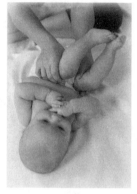

Divine Drops
page 79

Womb Wings
page 81

Apana
page 72

Corkscrew
page 74

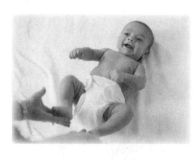 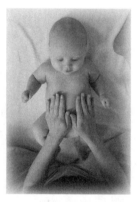 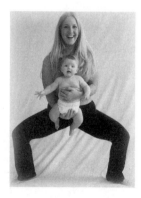

Chair Pose
page 47

Heart-Warm Touch
page 70

Divine Drops
page 79

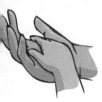

Daddy Series
• • • • • • • • • • • • •
Yoga for Head-Holders

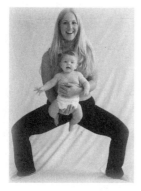

Divine Drops
page 79

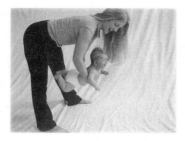

Womb Wings
page 81

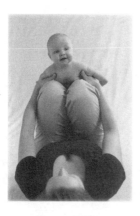
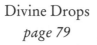

Super Baby
page 85

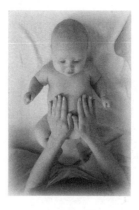

Heart-Warm Touch
page 70

Sleep Well Series

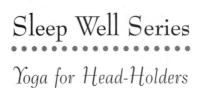

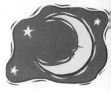

Yoga for Head-Holders

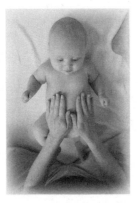

Heart-Warm Touch
page 70

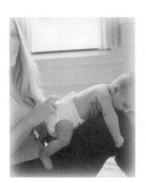

Dolphin
page 59

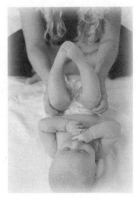

Apana
page 72

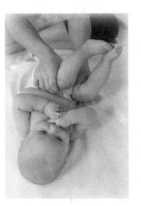

Corkscrew
page 74

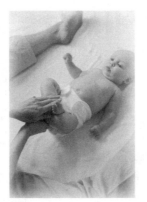

One Foot, Two Foot Lotus
page 83

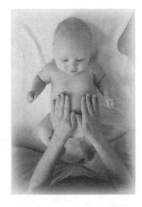

Heart-Warm Touch
page 70

Chapter 6

Yoga for the Almost Sitting

 Until I get more practice and I'm a little stronger, I'm an "almost-sitting baby" because if you took the pillows away or your hands off me, I would tip over immediately.

Older children and adults sit and stand during most of the day. Because it is so natural for us, we unconsciously encourage our babies to sit or stand before they are physically ready. An almost-sitting baby is working toward independent sitting. His abdominal muscles are just beginning to gain the strength necessary to lift and adequately support his torso. This stage of your baby's life lasts for a short period of time. It is literally weeks, in a lifetime of decades. It is important to allow the abdominal area to grow strong at its own pace before independent sitting, crawling, and walking take place.

Developing Your Baby's Core

Back problems in adults can occur when the lower back is working overtime in order to compensate for underdeveloped abdominal muscles. In yoga, we develop our abdominal muscles—our body's core strength—through *Uddiyana Bandha*. Uddiyana Bandha takes place when the lower stomach pulls back toward the spine, and the diaphragm lifts up toward the chest. The drawing back of the abdominal region contracts the belly, tilts or tucks the pelvis, and strengthens the lower back and torso. Yoga students with lingering lower back problems notice that their back problems disappear when their core is strengthened through Uddiyana Bandha. Your baby will develop Uddiyana Bandha naturally as he becomes an independent sitter. In this chapter, I Love You!, Rolio, Hip Circles, Padahasta, and Bridge Pose can help your baby's core flourish.

During this brief stage of your baby's life, when his core is not completely developed, always help support his abdominals and lower back when he is practicing his sitting postures by wrapping both your hands around his waist.

Introducing Tummy Time

When a baby lies on his belly it has a positive effect on his sitting posture. To offset the potential developmental delays caused by having your baby sleep on her back (an important precaution against to prevent SIDS), pediatricians encourage dedicated and supervised floor time for babies on their bellies, or Tummy Time. This practice helps a baby develop strength in the upper limbs, chest, and back, all of which are important for sitting and later crawling.

It is OK for your baby to grow into the pleasures of Tummy Time. The initial discomfort displayed when young infants are placed on their bellies may reflect their unease or fear of a new position. Some babies can get frustrated by the amount of effort it takes to lift their heavy heads up. You will find more about Tummy Time and an entire Developmental Series dedicated to Tummy Time in Chapter 7. But now is the time to begin to help your baby start incorporating Tummy Time into his schedule. Here are a few suggestions that work for many of my students.

Tummy Time Suggestions

- Cover a plastic birthing ball, or physioball, with a receiving blanket. Rest your baby's belly on top of the ball and blanket. Hold him securely as you gently roll him back and forth.

- Join your baby by coming down onto your own belly, or lie on your side to keep him amused (this is especially helpful when first beginning Tummy Time).
- Massage your baby's back while he lies across your thighs.
- Place a mirror at ground level in front of your baby so he can be entertained by his own image.
- Never leave your baby unattended during Tummy Time. And do not practice Tummy Time on a bed or changing table—you never know when babies may roll over!
- Tummy Time is best practiced on a clean floor area with one or two toys for your baby to play with.

What's Holding Your Baby?

Is your baby rolling and revealing other precursors to sitting and crawling? If you have noticed your baby pivoting 180 degrees in a semicircle, or sliding himself backward and pulling himself forward, you may feel safer keeping your baby in an infant car seat, swing, or activity saucer when you cannot hold him. In fact, life for parents would be difficult without these items when transporting a baby in the car, cooking dinner, and so on. However, these items are designed to confine a moving baby's activity, and their *overuse* restricts a baby's natural body movements and reduces positioning that is essential for a baby to become an independent mover, happy explorer, and active participant in play. Babies should not be confined unnecessarily in these supports for extended periods of time.

I work with many babies and can easily spot the ones who have jumpy seats at home. Babies love to bounce in these seats, but as an infant developmental movement specialist, I do not recommend them. The baby of one of my keen students was given a jumpy seat as a gift. After four days of use, she noticed that her baby was standing on his tiptoes rather than on a flat foot as he previously did. She packed the jumpy seat away and continued to bounce her baby, but now she bounces him on her lap while she sits on a big plastic birthing ball or physioball. I believe that jumping seats give babies a false sense of their center. After repeated use, a baby's legs to go into flexion when her feet hit the floor or any another surface, creating difficulties later on, when she begins to walk. Imagine how difficult it would be to stand or walk if every time your feet hit the floor they would bend and flex toward your chest. If your baby likes to bounce, practice the Yoga for Almost Crawlers collection (see Chapter 7) and share Hop Along Yogi, Divine Drops, and Lampa Season with him. Leave the jumpy seat at the store.

As you begin the yoga practice for almost-sitting babies:

- Gather a receiving blanket and a small baby toy or rattle.
- Find a full-length or decent-sized mirror to practice yoga near.
- Conduct the yoga practice on a changing table, with your undivided supervision, or on the carpet or a blanket.
- Play soft music and keep lighting subdued.
- Start with Belly Breathing (pages 24–25) or Ujjayi breathing (see page 51)
- End with a relaxation technique (pages 34-37).

If your baby is already sitting independently (that is, without props or your help), that's wonderful! He can continue to practice the *Yoga for the Almost Sitting* collection as well as continue onto our next chapter, *Yoga for Almost Crawlers*. A strong center or core is also necessary for the long reach forward a baby takes as crawling begins.

I Love You!

I Love You! Pose taught me how to fluctuate between being within my center and reaching out into the world. Notice how the movements in I Love You! expand my chest, filling me with prana or life force energy, and open my heart to receive and capture your love.

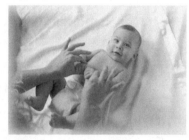

1. Position your baby on his back on a blanket with his feet nearest to you.

2. Place your thumbs into the palms of your baby's hands. Wrap your fingers around the outside of his hands.

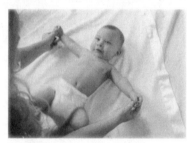

3. Mindfully repeat the words, "I Love You!" s-l-o-w-l-y as you and your baby perform the following movements together.

Sing & Do

I	Guide your baby's fists to his heart (top photo).
Love	Gently bring his fists and arms out to the sides (middle photo).
You	Guide the baby's fists to his heart and wiggle him side to side as he gives himself a hug (bottom photo). Repeat 3 to 5 times.

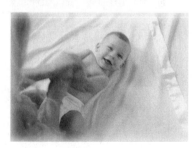

4. Share the Heart-Warm Touch with your baby.

Padahasta

. . . .

(Pada means foot and hasta means hand in Sanskrit)

Padahasta strengthens my digestive system and tones my legs. Try this pose with me anytime you want to help me relieve constipation or increase muscle tone in my legs.

1. Sit comfortably with your baby lying on her back in front of you with her feet closest to you.

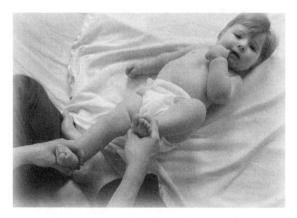

2. With your left hand hold your baby's right foot. Bring your thumb onto the sole or bottom of her foot. Let your other fingers rest on the topside of her foot.

3. Place your right thumb on the sole or bottom of your baby's left foot. Let your other fingertips rest on the topside of her left foot.

4. Pump your baby's knees in toward her chest in an alternating pumping fashion.

Sing & Do

Pa	Bring baby's right knee toward chest.
da	Extend baby's right leg away from chest.
Ha	Bring baby's left knee toward chest.
sta	Extend baby's left leg away from chest.
	Repeat 1 to 3 times.

Hip Circles

• • • • • • • • • • • •

Hip Circles help keep the fluidity of my little body flexible as the core muscles of my body develop in leaps and bounds.

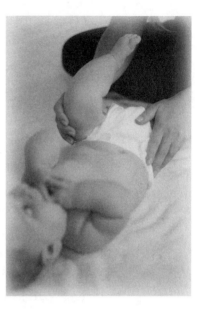

1. Position your baby on a blanket, on his back, with his feet nearest to you.

2. Place your right hand on top of your baby's left (nearest) hip.

3. Place your left thumb under your baby's right thigh with your fingers resting on top of his thigh.

4. Keep your right hand on his left hip to isolate the movement of his right leg.

5. With your left hand, draw a slow, clockwise circle with your baby's knee. This is done by bringing the flexed knee out to the side and then circling his knee in toward the center of his chest.

Sing & Do

Hip	Circle baby's right knee and leg clockwise.
Hip	Repeat clockwise circle.
Hooray!	Repeat clockwise circle.
Circle	Circle baby's right knee and leg counterclockwise.
Circle	Repeat counterclockwise.
Whee!	Repeat counterclockwise.

6. Switch sides and circle your baby's left knee using the Sing & Do Technique.

7. Share the Heart-Warm Touch with your baby and let him know how good exercise is for him.

Rolio

• • • • • •

Rolio gives my lower back and nearby organs a nice massage and helps me increase my whole body coordination. A good rhythm in Rolio can take the edge off of my fussiness. Try it and watch for my facial expressions to let you know how much you can speed up the rolling.

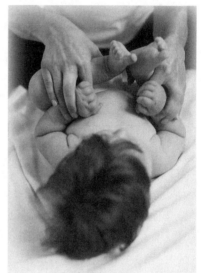

1. Position your baby on her back with your feet nearest to you. Using both of your hands, bring your baby's two hands together above her chest.

2. While continuing to hold your baby's hands together with one hand, use your dominant hand to bring her feet up into your hands one at a time.

3. Now your baby's hands and feet are held with your two hands. Place both of your thumbs behind the heels of her feet. Position your baby's wrists between your middle and index fingers. Your remaining fingers rest gently on top of her wrists (top photo).

4. Let the fun begin! Roll your baby's body from side to side as fast or as slow as she would like (bottom photo).

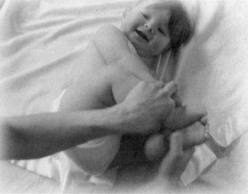

Sing & Do

Ro	Roll your baby to the left.
Li	Roll your baby to center.
O	Roll your baby to the right.
	Continue for 5 to 30 seconds.

Be sure to keep my head aligned with my heart. If it isn't, I need you to roll me slower.

5. Joyfully cheer and clap your baby's hands or feet together.

Kissy Feet

Even though my feet are so small, each foot contains over 7,200 nerve endings. Reflexologists believe that touching energetic points in my foot can improve the health of my organs, tissues, and nerve endings. Kissy Feet improves circulation in my legs, and also helps me feel the soles of my feet without the effort of standing.

1. Let your baby lie on his back with his feet nearest to you.

2. Place your thumbs on the outside of your baby's ankles.

3. Wrap your fingers along the inside of his ankles and lower legs.

4. Begin to clap his feet together.

5. Use a high-pitched voice and a drumlike tempo as you perform Sing & Do.

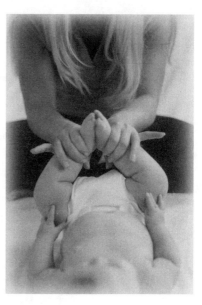

♪ ♪ Sing & Do

Kis-	Bring feet together.
sy	Pull feet apart quickly.
Feet	Bring feet together and pull apart quickly.
	Repeat 3 to 5 times.

6. Share your kisses with your baby's little feet!

7. Finish by stretching your baby's legs out long toward you.

Name Singing

Name Singing makes my self-esteem soar! I love my name and when big people sing it to me sweetly I know they love me. If you want my attention in a hurry, sing my name sweetly and I am yours!

1. Give your baby a warm smile. Take a deep breath, filling your lower belly, heart, and chest. When ready, exhale completely, releasing any tension.

2. At the top of your next inhale, begin to sing your baby's name in your sweetest, most angelic voice.

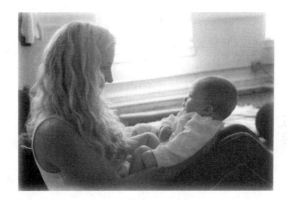

3. Observe your baby's reactions as you repeat it 3 to 5 times.

4. Applaud your baby as you joyfully connect with each other.

Additional Ways to Practice Name Singing

- If you have any pets or other children at home, try Name Singing to them too!
- Try using Name Singing in the car to help calm a baby.
- Name Sing all family members' names each morning.

Tushie Touches

·············

When I am on my belly and lift my head, I am strengthening the muscles that will eventually help me roll. As you continue to share Tushie Touches with me I will put weight on my arms, look around, and play. Tushie Touches are also good for stretching and toning my thighs.

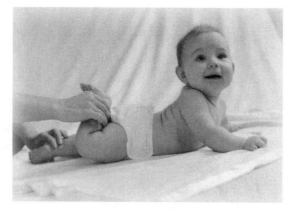

1. Sit comfortably with your legs crossed in front of you or in a V position.

2. Put your baby on his tummy on the blanket in front of you so that your baby's feet are nearest to you.

3. Cup your hands around your baby's lower legs with your fingertips facing in toward each other.

4. If your baby's knee is willing to bend; begin to bring his heel in toward his tushie. It is not necessary for your baby's heel to touch his tush today if it means using your strength to do so.

If my knee is stiff, hold my leg with less force and tell me to relax. Try this same leg again or switch to my other leg and come back to this leg later.

♪ ♪ ♪ ## Sing & Do

Tushie   Guide to your baby's right heel to his tush.
Touches   Lengthen your baby's right leg.
            Continue for 5 to 25 seconds.

Variation: Tushie Touches Toy

With your baby is lying on his belly, put a small toy on the floor between his hands. Notice if he begins to prop himself up on his forearms and belly. Once he can do so, his hands become free to play with the toy and he can engage in hand-to-hand play. This teaches your baby about body awareness and tactile exploration.

Bridge

●●●●●●●

When I am holding Bridge Pose with your loving assistance, I become aware of the strength in my legs, thighs, hips, and abdomen. Bridge Pose provides me with a feeling of connection between my pelvis and feet that will begin to support me in sitting and later standing.

1. Comfortably kneel, or sit with your legs in a V position.

2. Position your baby on her back crosswise in front of you with head near your right knee and her feet near your left knee.

3. Use your left hand to gently hold of the tops of your baby's feet. This will help keep her feet in place on the floor during Bridge.

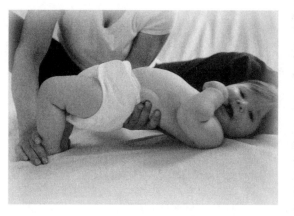

4. Slide your right hand, palm up underneath your baby's hips.

5. With your right palm lift your baby's hips about 3 inches from the floor.

YOUR BABY'S UPPER BACK AND SHOULDERS SHOULD REMAIN ON THE FLOOR DURING BRIDGE POSE.

♪ *Sing & Do*

Bridge Pose   Keep your baby's hips elevated.

6. Hold Bridge Pose for 5 seconds to 30 seconds or as long as your baby feels comfortable.

7. Slowly lower your hand that is under your baby's hip. This allows your baby's tush to once again rest on the floor.

8. Use both hands to bring your baby's knees up toward her chest (as in Apana, page 72) and then relax them down to the blanket.

Headstand

. . . .

Headstands benefit my entire nervous system and senses. With each headstand my brain receives a fresh supply of oxygen-rich blood so that I am can grow stronger and sleep better.

CAUTION: IF YOUR BABY IS ON MEDICATION, OR HAS CARDIAC PROBLEMS OR SEIZURES, CHECK WITH YOUR PHARMACIST OR PEDIATRICIAN TO SEEK THEIR PERMISSION BEFORE PLACING YOUR BABY INTO ANY INVERTED POSITIONS.

1. Consider having a full-length mirror nearby. It will give you both a great view of your baby's headstand and each other.

2. Sit with your legs together and stretched out in front of you.

3. Gently place your baby's back against your shins with his head by your feet. Your baby's spine should be aligned with the line between your legs.

4. Leave a few inches between your baby's head and your ankles. To create that gap, slide his feet toward you.

5. Firmly place your hands on the front of your baby's hips. This will keep him safely in place.

6. By bending your knees, slowly elevate your baby to a 45-degree angle from the floor. Hold this pose for 10 seconds. Gradually increase the time in small increments working up to a full minute.

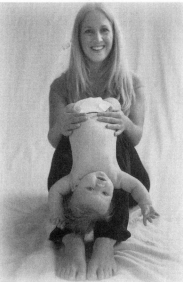

If I become uneasy in Headstand, immediately lower your legs and let me rest on my back, as described in steps 7 and 8.

7. When your baby sounds or looks ready to come out of the pose, slowly lower your legs to the floor.

8. Let your baby rest on his back for one minute. This rest is important for balancing the increased flow of energy and blood after a headstand.

One-on-One

As we do One-on-One our bodies move together as one and my sense of balance and moving through space improves. During One-on-One I like to imagine that I inspire your body movements to amplify the movements I am attempting to make. One-on-One can bring an important balance in all family relationships as we take turns giving and receiving, initiating and responding with love.

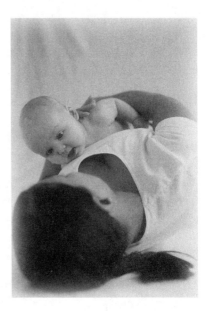

1. Sit with your feet on the floor and your knees bent into a 45-degree angle.

2. Hold your baby against your chest and slowly lie down. Keep your feet on the floor and knees angled.

3. Slide her so you're belly-to-belly with each other.

4. Relax with your baby as you find a similar breathing rhythm.

5. As your hands keep her secure, begin to initiate small rolling movements with your torso.

6. Let your baby inspire you as you increase the tempo of rolling.

7. Push from your feet to continue the One-on-One rolling of you and your baby for the next 30 to 60 seconds.

8. After 30 to 60 seconds of One-on-One, slow the tempo until you rest into stillness with her on your heart and belly. Relax as you prepare for Shavasana, our closing relaxation, or your next pose.

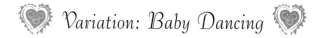 *Variation: Baby Dancing*

From Step 6, slowly come up into standing with your baby. Put on your favorite song and dance freely through the room while holding your baby. Explore moving side to side, up and down, and in spiral movements to the beat of the music. Let your baby inspire you, and continue for as long as you like.

Good Morning Series

· ·

Yoga for the Almost Sitting

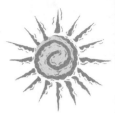

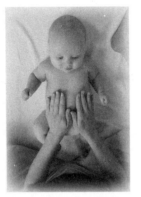

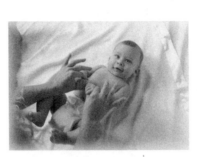

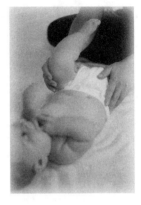

Heart-Warm Touch with Name Singing
pages 70, 101

I Love You!
page 95

Hip Circles
page 97

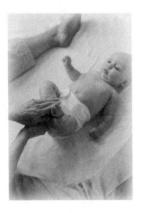

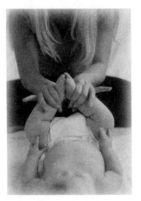

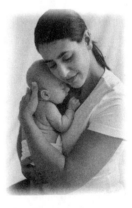

One Foot, Two Foot, Lotus
page 83

Kissy Feet
page 100

Scoop n' Hug
page 49

Developmental Play Series

· ·

Yoga for the Almost Sitting

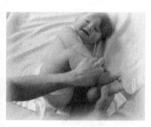

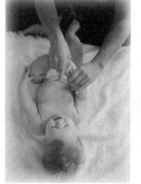

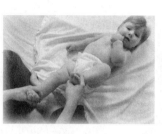

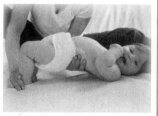

Rolio
page 98

Brain Builders
page 77

Padahasta
page 96

Bridge
page 104

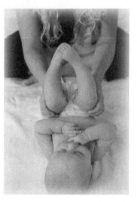

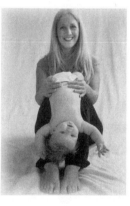

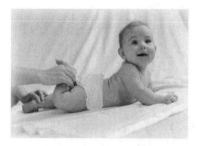

Apana
page 72

Headstand
page 106

Tushie Touches
page 102

Happy Baby Series

Yoga for the Almost Sitting

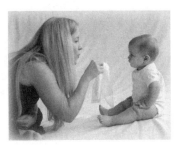

Belly Breathing
pages 24–25

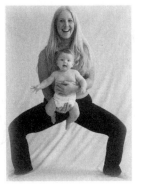

Divine Drops
page 79

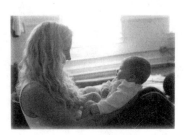

Name Singing
page 101

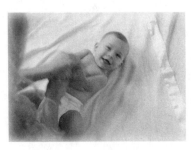

I Love You!
page 95

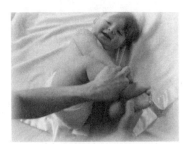

Rolio
page 98

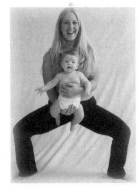

Divine Drops
page 79

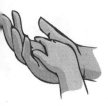

Daddy Series
· · · · · · · · · · · · · ·
Yoga for the Almost Sitting

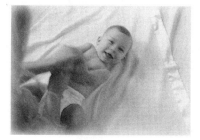

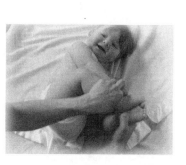

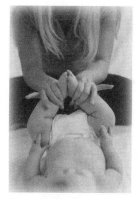

I Love You!
page 95

Rolio
page 98

Kissy Feet
page 100

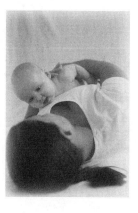

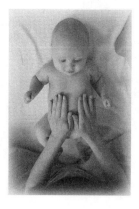

One-on-One
page 108

Heart-Warm Touch
page 70

Sleep Well Series

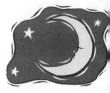

Yoga for the Almost Sitting

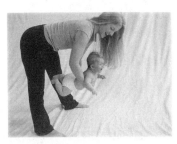

Womb Wings
page 81

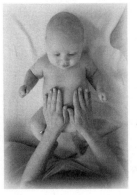

Heart-Warm Touch
page 70

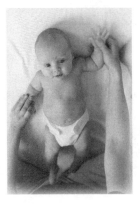

Twinkle
page 75

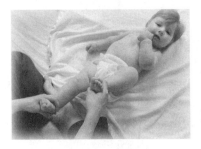

Padahasta
page 96

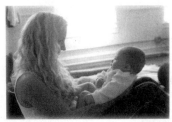

Name Singing
page 101

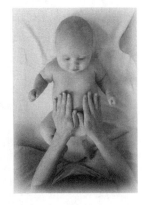

Heart-Warm Touch
page 70

Chapter 7

Yoga for Almost Crawlers

When you see me on my hands and knees rocking back and forth in a repetitive motion as if I am trying to launch myself into space, I am an almost-crawling baby.

A baby's umbilical cord is positioned on her belly and carries nutrients from her mother so the baby can grow and survive in the womb. Just as the umbilical cord connects a baby with its mother, the baby also connects its navel with gravity and Mother Earth. By putting your baby on his belly for Tummy Time you are facilitating the underlying connection your baby needs to make in relationship to gravity. Tummy Time nurtures abdominal strength, lumbar or lower back strength, and movement through space. Tummy Time also helps babies develop strong arms and necks, which they need to support their bodies in crawling. Once your baby realizes all the things that she can see and play with while resting on her tummy, it may become one her most favored positions as she learns to crawl. Crawling helps connect both halves of the brain and body. Studies show crawling can help reduce reading and communication difficulties later in childhood.

With yoga, you are spending time with your baby where your baby spends her time—on the floor. By doing so you send the message that you are willing to participate in her explorations. When you are fully present with your baby, she will show you how she loves to connect with you socially.

As an infant developmental movement educator, I want to share what happens after Tummy Time and before crawling so that you can follow your baby's progression of developmental movement every step of the way.

The Progression from Tummy Time to Crawling:

1. Tummy Time
2. Yoga's Table Pose (up on all fours)
3. Table rocking (a term to describe rocking back and forth on hands and knees)
4. Yoga's Downward Facing Dog
5. Pushing backward, moving away from what they want to go toward
6. Belly crawling
7. Crawling

When your baby is ready, she will lift your belly off the floor and come onto her hands and knees. This position mirrors yoga's **Table Pose**. Once in table pose, your baby may begin rocking back and forth repeatedly. I call this stage table rocking. **Table rocking** helps babies figure out where their limbs are in relationship to each other and in space. More important, table rocking also helps a baby register velocity of movement, balance, and spatial orientation.

Yoga's Downward Facing Dog Pose is instrumental in connecting and coordinating movements between a baby's lower and upper limbs to elevate her body in height. When babies are learning to walk, Downward Facing Dog becomes a transitional move to come up into standing.

Pushing backward to come toward something may seem frustrating, but many times you have to put the car in reverse before you can drive forward and get where you are going. A push from the upper limbs moves a baby backward. A reach of the upper limbs will bring a baby forward and into belly crawling.

Belly crawling is exactly that—crawling on the belly. As a baby begins to move forward on her belly you may notice the arm and leg on one side extend while the arm and leg on the opposite side flex. A baby starts to differentiate the between the right and left sides of her body during belly crawling. Sometimes belly crawling is known as the military or army crawl.

Crawling, more technically known as creeping, happens when babies want something out of reach and go after it on hands and knees. During crawling, babies reach forward with one arm as the opposite back knee pulls forward. The reach of the hand that extends through the baby's navel and pulls the diagonally opposite knee forward is believed to integrate both halves of the brain and body.

Yoga gives your baby the confidence and strength to move forward into crawling. This is such a fun time to start or continue yoga with your baby. She is willing to show you so much of her personality and absolutely loves to move and be played with.

Babies learn through play with toys and interactions with others. Try following the yoga poses in this book with your mothers group or play-group. This is the time when babies absolutely love to be around other babies. In fact one of the joys in my classes is to see a baby hug or kiss another baby. Everyone's heart melts at seeing how much these tender little beings just want to give and receive love.

Up until the recent past, a whole village or extended family would raise a baby. Nowadays, we expect one or two parents to do it alone. That's not healthy and can be stressful. Build a small community one person at a time or find one that's already established. If you don't have friends who have babies, you can call area organizations or visit www.ItsyBitsyYoga.com to find a trained and certified Itsy Bitsy Yoga facilitator, or connect with like-minded new parents in your area. You are not alone nor do you need to be.

As you begin yoga practice for almost-crawling babies:

- Gather a receiving blanket, a small baby toy, and ball.
- Practice on the carpet or a blanket.
- Play soft music.
- Start with Belly Breathing (pages 24–25) or Ujjayi breathing (see page 51).
- End with a relaxation technique (pages 34–37).

Toes to the Nose

* * * * * * * * * * * * * * * *

(level 1)

Toes to the Nose tends to move things around in my belly, helping me go poopie! As we do Toes to the Nose notice how super-flexible my hips and legs are. Yoga can help my body maintain flexibility throughout my life.

1. Sit comfortably with your baby lying on her back with her feet nearest you.

2. With your right hand grasp your baby's leg just above her left ankle. Rest your thumb on her calf and your first two fingers on her shin.

3. Guide your baby's toes to her nose.

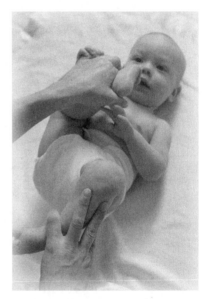

Please notice where my flexibility lessens so that we work together in yoga and in life. Knowing that you don't want to force any of my limbs means that you respect my wishes and body.

4. Tickle her nose with her toes.

5. In a playful voice sing "Toes to the Nose" and accentuate the "O" in the words "toes," "to," and "nose" as you continue with Sing & Do.

Sing & Do

Toes	Hold baby's left foot near her ankle.
to the	Bring baby's toes to the nose.
Nose	Tickle nose with toes.
	Repeat 3 to 5 times and look for your baby's reactions.

6. Switch sides and guide your baby's right toes to the her nose, repeating Sing & Do.

7. Thank your baby as you share Heart-Warm Touch with her legs and entire body.

Siddha Twistee

• • • • • • • • • • • • • •

Siddha Twistee helps strengthen and restore the muscles in between my ribs that I use in rolling, sitting, and—soon—crawling. Everything inside my belly feels so good when I twist in Siddha Twistee! Notice the peaceful look this pose brings to my face.

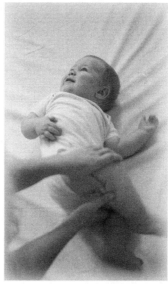

1. Have a small toy nearby.
2. Begin with your baby lying on his back with his feet nearest you.
3. Wrap your hands around his upper thighs.
4. Bring his legs knees slightly toward his chest.
5. Follow the appropriate next step based on the present position of your baby's head.

If your baby is looking away from you:

- Slowly turn your baby's knees toward the floor in the direction opposite to his stare.
- Hold for 3 to 5 seconds.

If your baby is looking at you:

- With both hands gently turn your baby's stacked knees to the right.
- Use your top hand to keep his knees in position.
- Remove your bottom hand from under your baby and hold your baby's toy for him to look in the opposite direction.
- Entice your baby to look to his left by positioning his toy 8 inches diagonally above the left side of his body.
- Hold for 3 to 5 seconds.

Sing & Do

Siddha	Bring baby into pose.
Twistee	Hold pose for 3 to 5 seconds.
	Repeat 1 to 3 times.

6. Use your baby's toy to direct his head and gaze to the opposite direction and switch sides. Repeat the Sing & Do Technique.

7. Extend baby's legs and feet down toward you.

8. Share the Heart-Warm Touch (page 70) or Here & Now pose (page 58) with your baby!

9. Tuck your baby's toy away behind you so he can remain focused on you and yoga.

Lampa Season

(Lampa is the Sanskrit word for Jump!)

Lampa season is one way that we can merrily bounce happiness into any day of the year! This is a great pose to do with me when I can use a little joy or movement to melt away the frustration of wanting to crawl!

1. Sit in a comfortable cross-legged position.

2. Place your hands under your baby's armpits.

3. Place your baby on top of one knee in an upright sitting position. Her feet will be dangling toward the floor as you support her body upright with your hands.

4. Slowly start to bounce both knees and baby. Enliven the pace to your baby's liking.

5. Add the Sing & Do Technique, jumping baby up from one knee to the other as cued with the change of seasons.

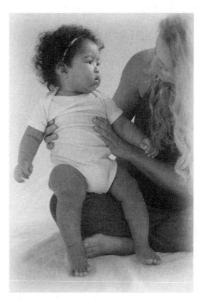

Sing & Do

Lampa	Bounce baby on left knee.
Spring	Bounce baby
Lampa	Bounce baby
Spring	Bounce baby
Lampa	Bounce baby
Spring	Bounce baby
Showers!	Lift baby up high and over to your right knee!
Lampa	Bounce baby on right knee.
Summer	Bounce baby

Lampa	Bounce baby
Summer	Bounce baby
Lampa	Bounce baby
Summer	Bounce baby
Sun!	Lift baby up high and over to your left knee!

Lampa	Bounce baby on left knee.
Fall	Bounce baby
Lampa	Bounce baby
Fall	Bounce baby
Lampa	Bounce baby
Fall	Bounce baby
Leaves!	Lift baby up high and over to your right knee!

Lampa	Bounce baby on right knee.
Winter	Bounce baby
Lampa	Bounce baby
Winter	Bounce baby
Lampa	Bounce baby
Winter	Bounce baby
Snow!	Lift baby up high and into your arms!

6. Clap with your baby; you're both doing a great job!

Butterfly

· · · · · · · · · ·

The ring shape of my legs in Butterfly makes for a very stable base for me to sit upon. In traditional adult yoga, this pose is called "Baddha Konasana" or Bound Angle Pose.

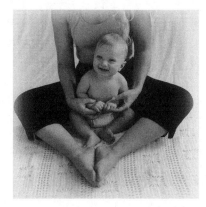

1. Sit with your legs in a modified Bound Angle Pose or *Baddha Konasana* from yoga. Loosely bring your knees outward and turn your feet inward. Your legs should form a loose diamond shape with the soles of your feet facing each other.

2. Let the soles of your feet come apart or extend them further away from you to create enough space for your baby to sit in.

3. Invite or help him into the center of the diamond shape. Let him sit facing away from you with his back to your chest.

4. Bring the soles of his feet as close together as he'd like.

5. With your hands, invite your baby's legs to make flapping movements like butterfly wings.

Sing & Do

Butter   Lift baby's knees up high.
Fly   Let baby's knees float down.
             Repeat 3 to 5 times.

6. Finish with an warm, embracing hug.

Baby Plank

In Baby Plank it looks like I am at the top of a push-up. As I learn to crawl, I can feel the palms of my hands starting to open as I strengthen my upper body and my developing arms. I can also feel a sense of power growing in my belly because Plank Pose engages and tones my abdominal area. With strength in both my belly and arms I am one step closer to lifting my belly off the ground and crawling.

1. Sit with your legs extended on the floor in a V position. Put your baby's small soft toy on the floor between your ankles.

2. Support your baby in a standing position and place her back against your chest.

3. Place one hand on your baby's chest and the other across her thighs.

4. Extend your arms out in front of you to bring your baby forward.

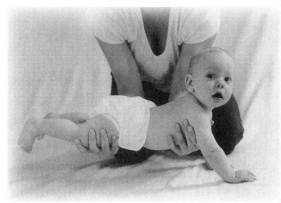

5. Continue to bring your baby's front side into a position parallel to the floor without reaching the blanket. It should look like she's flying, one of her arm's lengths above the blanket.

6. Let your baby's arms extend and reach down to the floor or her toy. Eventually your baby's palms will open, allowing her to support her upper body.

HINT: If she needs some encouragement to reach for the floor, bring her attention to the small toy you earlier placed near your ankles.

7. Hold for 5 to 20 seconds, allowing your baby time to build strength and trust.

8. Repeat once.

Bala

· · · · ·

(Bala is the Sanskrit word for Child)

 Bala pose helps me discover my knees, and that's superhelpful now that I want to crawl and pull myself up into standing. When you help me kneel-stand as in Bala Pose, we prepare the longest bones in my body, the femurs, for good posture and balance.

1. Have a ball nearby and kneel behind your baby as he rests on his stomach.

2. Use your hands to tuck your baby's knees slightly under his body.

3. Move yourself forward to comfortably include your baby within your kneeling stance so that the insides of your legs are hugging the outside of his.

4. Slide your right hand under your baby's belly.

5. Draw his hips back toward you.

6. With your right hand lift your baby's chest into upright. He is now in a supported kneel-standing position.

♪ Sing & Do

Bala	Place ball in front of your baby and keep it snug with your knees.
Ba	Help drum baby's right hand on ball.
la	Help drum baby's left hand on ball.
Ba	Help drum baby's right hand on ball.
la	Help drum baby's left hand on ball.
	Continue for 5 to 15 seconds.

7. Bring your baby out of kneel-standing by lifting him up and holding him close to your heart.

Hop Along Yogi

(Yogi refers to a yoga student)

Hop Along Yogi is an all-time favorite of mine. If you happen to be doing Hop Along Yogi when our friends or family are around, let me face them so everyone can share my smile. Sometimes when Mom and Dad want me to smile for pictures, they bounce up and down singing the words to Hop Along Yogi.

1. Sit with your legs extended together in front of you.

2. Sit your baby on your thighs facing you or looking our into the room

3. Wrap your hands around her body.

4. Begin to bounce your baby by bending and lifting your knees up from the floor and then straightening your legs down quickly. The verses of the song will vary the pace of the exercise.

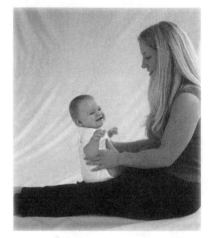

Sing & Do

Hop along yogi	Bounce legs in a slow to medium pace.
Hop along yogi	Bounce legs in a slow to medium pace.
Hop along yogi	Bounce legs in a slow to medium pace.
Real, real slow!	Bounce legs in a slow to medium pace.
Hop along yogi	Bounce legs in a medium to fast pace.
Hop along yogi	Bounce legs in a medium to fast pace.
Hop along yogi	Bounce legs in a medium to fact pace.
Real, real fast!	Bounce legs in a medium to fast pace.

Hop along yogi	Bounce legs in a fast pace.
Hop along yogi	Bounce legs in a fast pace.
Hop along yogi	Bounce legs in a fast pace.
Here we go!	Lean or roll back with baby, or lift your baby high with your arms.

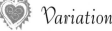 Variation: Hop Along Name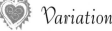

Replace the word "yogi" with your baby's name and repeat step 4. For instance, "Hop along Matthew, Hop along Matthew, Hop along Matthew, Real, real slow," and so on.

Special You Song

The Special You Song teaches me the names of my body parts and where they are located. It also brings awareness to the seven major energy centers, or chakras, of a body. After all, it's the prana, or life force, moving through our body that helps to make us special!

1. The Special You Song is easy to sing and the beat is similar to "If you're happy and you know it, clap your hands."

2. Sit comfortably. The preferred position for your baby is lying down, but if he wants to sit in your lap right now, that's fine too.

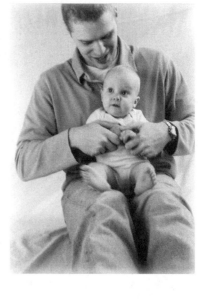

Sing & Do

If you're special and you know it, touch your head!
Your hands touch the top of your baby's head.

If you're special and you know it, touch your eyes!
Your hands lightly touch your baby's eyebrows.

If you're special and you know it, touch your throat!
Your hands touch just below his throat.

If you're special and you know it, touch your heart!
Place your hands over his heart.

If you're special and you know it, touch your tummy!
Place your hands on his tummy.

If you're special and you know it, touch your belly button!
Place your hands about an inch below his belly button.

If you're special and you know it, touch your legs!
Your hands touch baby's thighs.

If you're special and you know it, touch your feet!
Hold baby's feet with your hands.

You're special and you know it 'cause your body is here to show it!
Caress your baby with a steady, smooth stroke of your hand from head to toe.

You are special and you know it—Namaste!
Place the palms of your hands together in front of your heart. Bow to honor
yourself and your baby.

💗 Variation: Special Finds 💗

Help your baby's hands touch his body parts in the Special You Song as
you sing to him.

Kicky Cobra

 In Kicky Cobra I feel I am swimming, and I'm strengthening my lower body awareness and power. Kicky Cobra is something that I will be trying to master on my own in the coming months.

1. Sit with your legs in a V position.

2. Place your baby facing away from you and on his belly.

3. With both hands hold your baby's lower legs, midway between your baby's knees and ankles.

4. Begin to flutter his feet in an alternating fashion. Repeat the following words and accentuate the "k" sound.

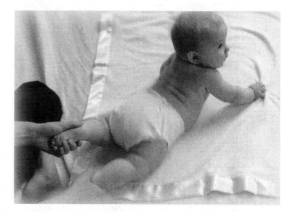

Sing & Do

Kick	Flutter kick baby's right foot.
Kick	Flutter kick baby's left foot.
Kick	Flutter kick baby's right foot.
Kick	Flutter kick baby's left foot.
K-i-c-k-y	Quickly flutter kick baby's feet continuously.
C-o-b-r-a!	Quickly flutter kick baby's feet continuously.
	Repeat 1 to 3 times.

Guppy

Guppy Pose expands my chest and lungs while relaxing my neck and upper and middle back. It also helps to boost my immune system. If you suspect I may be catching a cold, do Guppy Pose with me often.

1. Sit comfortably with your legs in a V shape.

2. Place your baby on his back across your thighs, with his shoulders resting over the top of your right thigh. It is important that both of his shoulders are resting on top of your thigh.

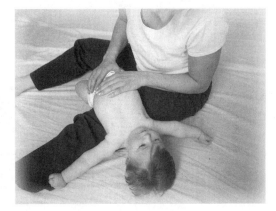

3. Place your left hand on his belly so he feels secure.

4. Help your baby relax his head back toward the floor.

5. Place your right hand behind his head for support if needed.

Sing & Do

Guppy Pose   Work up to holding Guppy Pose for 45 seconds. Start with 5
Guppy Pose   seconds and add 5-second increments until you reach 45
Guppy Pose   seconds or your baby's maximum.

6. To help your baby out of Guppy Pose, place your right hand behind your baby's head and slowly bring him to a sitting position or into your arms for a great big hug!

Good Morning Series

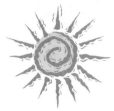

Almost Crawlers

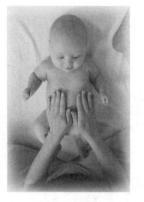

Heart-Warm Touch
page 70

Rolio
page 98

Siddha Twistee
page 121

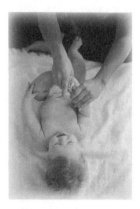

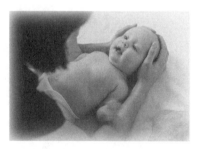

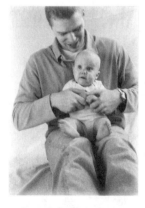

Brain Builders
page 77

Baby Planet
page 78

Special You Song
page 130

Tummy Time Series

· ·

Almost Crawlers

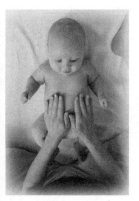

Heart-Warm Touch
page 70

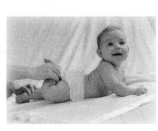

Tushie Touches
page 102

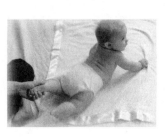

Kicky Cobra
page 132

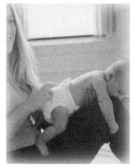

Dolphin
page 59

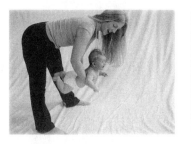

Womb Wings
page 81

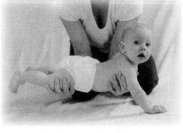

Baby Plank
page 126

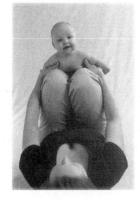

Super Baby
page 85

Happy Baby Series

Almost Crawlers

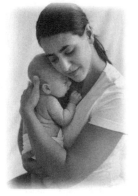

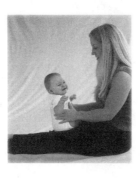

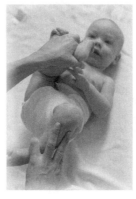

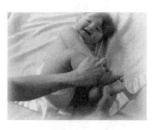

Scoop n' Hug
page 49

Hop Along Yogi
page 129

Toes to the Nose
page 119

Rolio
page 98

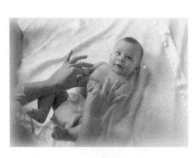

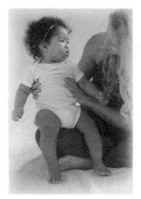

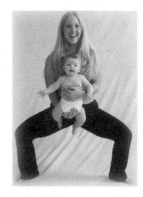

I Love You!
page 95

Lampa Season
page 123

Divine Drops (level 2
Head-Holder version)
page 79

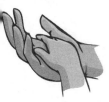

Daddy Series
• • • • • • • • • • • • • • •
Almost Crawlers

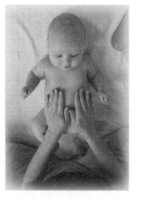

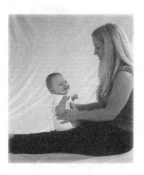

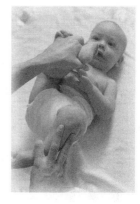

Heart-Warm Touch
page 70

Hop Along Yogi
page 129

Toes to the Nose
page 119

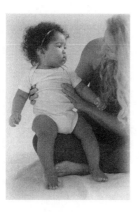

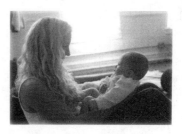

Lampa Season
page 123

Name Singing
page 101

Sleep Well Series

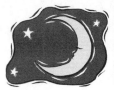

Almost Crawlers

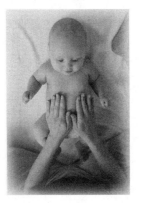

Heart-Warm Touch
page 70

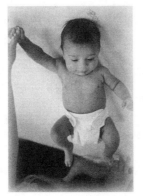

Tiny Tugs
page 57

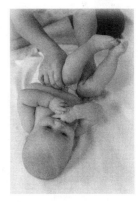

Corkscrew
page 74

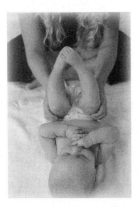

Apana
page 72

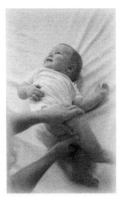

Siddha Twistee
page 121

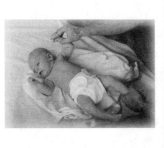

Here & Now
page 58

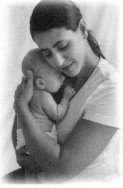

Scoop n' Hug
page 49

Chapter 8

Tots Yoga Fundamentals

 You know I am ready for Tots Yoga as soon as I begin crawling. Tots Yoga helps me move, grow strong, and have fun with you! I'll be doing more and more yoga on my own, and we are both much more active with the Tots Yoga.

Yoga for mobile babies is a mobile practice. We'll breathe, sing, move, sit, crawl, hop, jump, run, and relax. A baby is better at expressing herself with her body than with words. To inhibit a baby's movement is to inhibit an important way she expresses herself. Show your baby that you are willing to go with the flow and listen to her body language. I like to think of yoga as a time for babies to learn the gifts of a healthy, moving body and for us to witness them blossoming.

If you are just starting this book, or are new to yoga, now is a perfect time for you and your baby to begin. If you have already shared yoga with your baby, you'll be amazed at how your baby's yoga practice changes and develops over the next few weeks and months. Your baby's excitement for independence and yoga will grow. In fact, you may catch your baby attempting to do many of the yoga postures on her own. As you call out a pose's name, pause and see your baby attempting to bring herself into position. Pretty soon your baby's attempts and yoga practice will pay off. Your baby will be doing yoga on command, especially as she starts walking.

Clear the Space

If you've been to a yoga studio, you may have noticed how clutter free and empty the room was. With limited outer distractions people feel safe and comfortable going within themselves. A clutter-free studio is symbolic of a clutter-free mind. Practice yoga in a childproof and simple space. The ideal place for you to share yoga with your baby is your bedroom or any area of the house that is empty or relatively clutter free. At this point in a baby's yoga practice, toys can become a distraction. When you clear toys from your baby's yoga space, your baby can focus more on you and yoga.

Unlike yoga practice with an infant, the entire room now becomes the yoga mat. One of the ways to succeed in doing yoga with a mobile baby is not to think that the poses need to take place on a two-by-three-foot blanket.

Adult practitioners of Itsy Bitsy Yoga need to clear both physical and mental space before doing yoga. If you have trouble letting go of mental to-do lists or worries, think of leaving them someplace where you can pick them up later if you choose. Leave the mental to-do list or let worries rest on a desk, not in between you and your child. Adapt the mind-clearing practice below to suit you. It will help prepare you mentally.

Mantra

*"When I am focused on my baby,
my baby is focused on me."*

Clear Your Mind

Invite yourself to close your eyes and gaze inward, toward the tip of your nose. Relax your bottom jaw. Feel your breath flowing in and out freely and without effort. Sit for five complete breath cycles of inhalation and exhalation.

Relax into the comfort of your love and your baby's love. If your baby starts to make a few sounds, hear her as if she's an angel speaking. Become aware of the thoughts that float through your mind. Allow each and every thought to float away, like clouds on a beautiful summer day. As you release the extraneous thoughts that may dwell in your mind, you are allowing something new to reveal itself to you.

Feel as if there is nothing to do but be present with your breath, your baby, and an empty mind. Know that this time is special and just for you and your baby. Be here for as long as you'd like. As you slowly open your eyes, allow some of your awareness to remain inward.

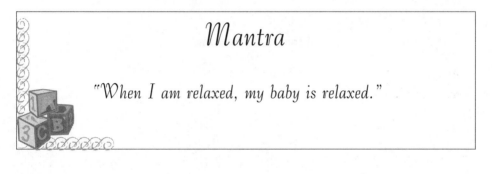

Mantra

"When I am relaxed, my baby is relaxed."

Fascinations

After you have eliminated the distractions and clutter, your baby may find a fascination during yoga. If a baby becomes fascinated with an object or body part, it is OK. Can you see things as he does? Be patient and give your baby a minute to finish exploring what he finds so interesting before resuming yoga. This communicates that you believe his curiosity is important.

Try moving with your baby if he chooses to explore. By staying with him, you regain his interest and move into the starting position for your next pose. After all, the entire room is a mobile baby's yoga mat.

Dressing for Yoga

Comfortable clothing that does not inhibit movement is ideal for yoga. Yoga is best practiced barefoot and without socks. Remove your baby's socks and shoes as you begin.

Props

The following props are helpful as you practice yoga with your tot:
- Yoga or exercise mat
- Full-length mirror
- Doll or stuffed animal that can move into yoga poses

Yoga Mat

If you have a yoga mat, great, bring it our during every practice. It helps your baby know it is time for yoga. As a baby grows, she'll start bringing out the mat to let you know that she wants to do yoga now. Also, the yoga mat provides a baby's hands and feet with a great sensory experience. (If you don't have a yoga mat, that's fine, you can still have a wonderful yoga practice.)

Mirror

When your baby was smaller, you used to watch your baby's reactions and positioning. Now that changes. Between six and nine months, a baby begins to realize that his face in a mirror is a reflection. Notice how a baby is now full of expressions and smiles at the reflection. This is when a baby begins to associate positive feelings and happiness with his own reflection in a mirror. Yoga can help a baby feel confident about his appearance and body from an early age.

Doll

When I teach tots yoga, babies always preview the pose we are working on. To do this at home use a doll or stuffed animal with movable limbs to demonstrate the tots yoga poses for a baby. Try to use the same doll every time you practice.

Fourteen-month-old Audrey started moving her baby doll into yoga poses, too. Twenty-three-month-old Chloe would treat her brand-new little sister, Kira, to yoga. Chloe is able to perform Heart-Warm Touch and Tiny Tugs with little Kira.

Preparing for Yoga Practice

Babies love paper! If this book is open and lying next to you, chances are your baby's heart will be set on playing with it! To avoid this, learn one or two poses at a time. As you first practice the poses, do so with a doll or have someone read you the directions while you and your mobile baby do yoga together. Another option is to put this book into a clear cookbook holder. This allows you to keep the book open next to you and your baby.

Mantra

Mornings are for learning.

If you are thinking about spending twenty minutes or so learning yoga with your baby, then do it in the morning. Mornings are when your baby is ready to stay focused and learn new things like yoga. Once you both have learned the poses you can practice at any time of day.

Ultimately it is best to teach your baby poses when she is well rested and fed.

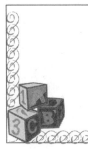

Mantra

Bedtime is for routines.

Yoga helps a mobile baby transition to sleep. It is a great time to practice the poses that you and your baby have learned. The Sleep Well Series at the end of each chapter highlights the poses that work especially well before bed. It is also helpful to use a softer voice when winding your baby down for the night.

When to Practice Yoga

With a mobile tot, long gone are the days of sitting in one spot and doing twenty to thirty minutes of yoga. Set your expectations to complete one to five poses each time. (Morning or bedtime is best for holding a baby's attention.) When you fine-tune the time of day and yoga series you choose to facilitate with your baby, the amount of distractions will lessen.

Yoga can be on the go, one Magic Pose to rid your baby of fussiness, a series to help her sleep through the night, or an entire chapter for a morning Bond & Be Well routine.

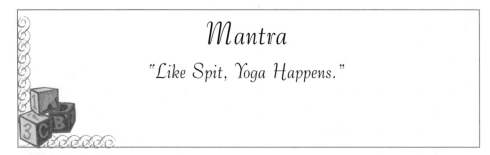

Mantra

"Like Spit, Yoga Happens."

Start to think of yoga as something that just happens anytime, anywhere. In your baby's mind yoga can happen anytime, not just between ten and ten-thirty on Monday, Wednesday, and Friday. As you become familiar with the poses, practice one here and one there. Perhaps you share a total of seven yoga poses with your almost-walking baby through the course of the day. For instance, Bridge Pose on the diaper table, Tree Pose when you are putting his shoes on, Lampa when you need to shift his focus, Down Dog in the living room, Clappy Happy Namaste before or after lunch, and Hop Along Yogi when you want him to be happy. See how it works? Yoga anytime, anywhere!

When practicing yoga try not to have an audience unless it is a parent. The exception is when a baby demonstrates a specific yoga pose on her own initiative. Having an audience is great then, because babies love the applause and attention. Seventeen-month-old Nolan would cut his pose short so he could come join us in clapping, cheering, and smiling for him.

As You Begin

To get me centered, continue to begin my yoga practice with Heart-Warm Touch (detailed on page 70), because I associate this touch with the good feelings of relaxation, comfort, and yoga. It's so nice to have a predictable pattern. It makes it easier for me to learn and boosts my confidence too!

Positioning

You and your baby's positioning will inevitably change several times during the session. If your baby crawls or walks off, don't get frustrated. Instead, re-engage him or bring him into the next posture. Mobile babies are fully aware of their surroundings and can't wait to touch, feel, and see everything. When your baby becomes familiar with the words in the posture's Sing & Do Technique you can repeat the Sing & Do words in order to have your baby join you in the pose. Remember, babies love yoga. A twenty-one-month-old student, Sasha, put herself into Fish Pose and said "Happy! Happy!" Her mother and I melted.

Tots like more freedom, so I've responded with Show Baby How and Baby's Turn techniques to complement the Sing & Do Technique.

Show Baby How

This is a great opportunity for you to do a little yoga! Approach it the way you want your baby to approach yoga and movement, with excitement and animation. Use a doll or your body to demonstrate the yoga pose. One-year-olds are great mimickers and love to see what you have to show them or what's coming up next for them. Remember, their minds are searching for patterns, and each time you lead them somewhere and then it happens, it's wonderful for them! I guess babies feels like adults do when we ask someone to do something for us and they do. During Show Baby How, the baby is invited to watch and study the shape of the pose, allowing her time to process what to do when it is Baby's Turn.

Baby's Turn

A baby who receives encouragement will soon begin to take more responsibility for her yoga practice. You'll really see how much she loves yoga! During Baby's Turn, stage 1, a parent or caregiver helps to facilitate a movement or pose. In stage 1 of Baby's Turn, babies work toward performing a pose or movement independently. During Baby's Turn it is important that you stay engaged and return to Sing & Do and Show Baby How as much as is necessary. Stage 2 is considered an intermediate version and uses minimal, if any, adult assistance. As with any sport, it takes time to learn how to play and feel confident. It is likely to take five or more practice sessions for a baby to respond in the Baby's Turn, stage 2 versions. Some poses will be mimicked independently more quickly than others. If after practicing a pose on five separate occasions your baby isn't responding to Baby's Turn, try to enliven and mix together Show Baby How and Baby's Turn. Remember, you can incorporate a baby's favorite stuffed animal or doll into the yoga poses. Stick with it and watch what takes place as your baby and her yoga practice grow.

Baby Pace

If we want to see our baby's sincerest movements and ways of being we need to slow down into the "baby pace." If you are not following the pace your baby sets, it's like trying to see an ant moving about on the side of the road while you're jogging along focused on getting your three miles in. Impossible! As you move together, see the world through the eyes of your baby, follow his pace, and see where he leads you. Baby pace is very important during Baby's Turn.

Babies are like very old photocopiers—they process very slowly. For this reason, leave a little time between poses (30 to 60 seconds is good). This allows time for him to integrate what he is learning or to try yoga movements independently. Watch for a baby to show you the yoga movements that feel good to his body. Be careful, though: leaving too much time can give some babies the opportunity to engage with something other than yoga.

Dealing with an Escaping Baby

Moving in and out of set spaces and activities is healthy and natural for babies. If your baby crawls off during yoga practice, it's OK. I simply follow the baby. When a baby is crawling or standing somewhere it's because that's where she wants to be, so let her be there and bring the yoga to her. Keep calm and playfully join your baby where she is. Follow your baby's body and mind. How can you take what has her attention and incorporate yoga into it?

Repetition and Learning

Babies thrive on repetition. Hearing the same rhymes and doing the same movements over and over again is how your baby learns them. No matter how poorly you sing, your baby will be a captive audience. The voice of a parent is a baby's favorite voice. Even if you're bored, he's not. Repetition develops memory and comprehension. The more animated you can become the more your baby will focus on what you have to show him.

Mirroring Back to Your Child

Reflect your joy in your baby's accomplishment to your baby. Reflecting acknowledges, informs, and illuminates. You may notice your baby showing you yoga outside the confines of your routine practice. When she does a pose or something close to it, tell her "Very good." Then mirror what her pose looked like, and call out the posture name.

One dad, Andrew, told me that out of the blue his son Lucas began doing Lampa. Lucas was even trying to say "Lampa," and his parents were greatly impressed with the positive impact yoga had on their nonvocal baby in just three classes. Andrew applauded him and repeated the pose's name for Lucas to hear. He took it one step further too: he did Lampa for Lucas to see! They smiled and felt connected with each other through yoga.

Customized Relaxation

If your baby is willing to let you close your eyes and practice a nonmoving relaxation technique as in Chapter 3, that's great! But if not, choose from this list of ways to relax and invite your baby to mimic you.

- Put on whatever music relaxes you and listen quietly while treasuring your baby.
- Take a relaxing bath with your baby or with your baby nearby.
- Go for a leisurely walk outdoors or explore nature with your baby.
- Go for a massage or give one to your baby.
- Practice yoga for yourself and have your baby watch you. Invite your wise little baby to listen to the words and thoughts that come to you.

Chapter 9

Yoga for Crawlers

Crawling is an exercise for my mind and body. As my limbs move in an alternating fashion, and my brain and body integrate, future learning has a solid foundation to build upon. Crawling also lets me move efficiently to the people, places, and things I want to explore which keep my spirit happy!

Crawling officially occurs when a baby reaches with one hand as the diagonally opposite knee lifts off the floor to follow the hand's reach. For the first time, crawlers can move about and take hold of what their hearts desire.

As your baby begins to crawl, create a safe space for him to explore. As long as a baby is safe, we should not impede his desire to explore his surroundings or to get somewhere. A baby's vehicle is his four-limbed body just as your vehicle is your four-wheeled car. Imagine you're driving your car and you end up hitting red light after red light, stop sign after stop sign, or a few dead ends every time you try to get somewhere. Eventually, you would simply lose your motivation to move at all. The same happens to babies as they get told "No, don't touch that," "Stop, don't go there," "Come back here," and "No!"

Give babies the freedom to crawl during their yoga practice so they can learn how to move in and out of activities and circumstances. This sets healthy boundaries for children. Giving crawling babies freedom to explore helps them know they can be where they want to be. Movement is a gift. It is something that parents and babies should feel good about doing together. Babies need to receive as much comfort from moving as they do from eating their favorite foods. If we had "comfort moves" instead of, or in addition to, "comfort foods," would it help lessen the alarming obesity rates in our children and adolescents?

If your baby crawls off during yoga practice, it's OK. Remain calm, she'll continue with yoga in a moment. When your baby crawls off, playfully meet her where she is and continue with yoga. One technique I use is to lovingly chase and catch them. Try moving into Ring Around the Yogi (described on page 157) so you can playfully go to her and resume yoga practice. Another technique is the Sing & Do. If you sing the words to a baby's favorite yoga poses, she may crawl back to you very quickly. Also, many of the Magic Poses in this book are great ways to reengage your exploring baby into yoga. If you give up repeatedly when your baby crawls off before you are done, does that mean that you are saying it's OK to quit?

Other, less spoken of, benefits of crawling are a healthy lower back and a strong sense of leg musculature. Because crawling is so good for physical and intellectual development, I encourage parents everywhere to let their babies be on the floor and master that activity before standing. In time a baby's body will progress naturally into different levels, including kneel-standing, squatting, and cruising.

Yoga can help crawlers feel connected to their parents during a time when separation anxiety becomes a real problem. To comfort your baby in your absence, show your baby's other primary caregivers how to do the Daddy Series or any of the yoga poses your baby loves. Yoga helps both working and stay-at-home parents deepen the bond with their children in short periods of time. And because infant massage becomes increasingly difficult with a baby on the go, yoga may be just the activity for a mobile baby who used to be massaged often.

In teaching parent and child yoga to thousands of mobile babies and toddlers, I witness parents' desire to maintain and grow their sense of connection with their babies who can crawl, walk, or push the parent away. It is of even greater importance for a child to know that every time he turns around, a loving parent or caregiver will be there for him. The treasure of being there for each other lasts a lifetime.

Introducing the Parent & Baby Loop

The Parent & Baby Loop is designed in part to help ease the challenge of letting a moving baby go one way while you want him to go another way. Through my Parent & Baby Loop method, I give parents an energetic way to loop in with each other always and easily.

How to Practice the Parent & Baby Loop

Take several deep breaths. Place your left hand over your solar plexus, which is located between your lower ribs, and your right hand over your navel. Feel connected with yourself. Gaze softly at your baby. If your baby is on your lap or next to you, place one hand on him. The breath is what connects you, so keep breathing. By being open to and aware of the space that exists between parent and child, you can remain in a loop, or connected, almost as if the umbilical cord were still attached. Slowly move your hands to a resting position away from your baby and body and still feel the sense of a clear, energy-filled tube connecting you and your little one, as if you are holding his long, invisible hand.

After you have been away from your baby for several hours, the Parent & Baby Loop and yoga are nice ways to reconnect. Even if you're with your baby all day, the time you spend doing yoga together feels special. It's best to practice yoga daily or at least three times per week. The time you spend doing yoga with your baby is truly quality time for you both. Many adults come to yoga class so that they have quality time for themselves. The practice of yoga is very centering for both you and your baby. When yoga is practiced wholeheartedly, students can begin to receive insights into who they are as parents and as people. And you'll glimpse the pearl of your child's true nature as it unfolds.

As you begin the yoga practice for crawlers

- Clear the space.
- Gather a handkerchief, lightweight scarf, or pinwheel for the Baby Blow.
- Put any nearby small toys away.
- When necessary, consider demonstrating the pose to your tot using a doll or stuffed animal.
- Find a full-length or decent-sized mirror to help you see your tot's reactions.
- Play soft music.
- Start with Belly Breathing (pages 24–25) and the Heart-Warm Touch (page 70).
- End with any of the relaxation techniques described on pages 34–37.

Baby Blow

 I naturally breathe in a yogic fashion, through my nose. Baby Blow builds upon this natural exhaling, bringing intent and mindfulness into my breathing activity. Baby Blow helps me be calm, centered, and focused.

1. Have a couple of tissues, opened napkins, or handkerchiefs nearby.
2. Sit comfortably on the floor or in a chair.
3. Invite your baby to sit facing you.

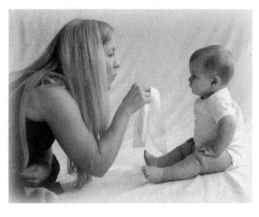

Show Baby How:

4. Dangle a tissue in your hand between you and your baby.
5. Take a deep, long breath in, filling your lungs with fresh air and life.
6. Exhale through your nose and move slightly toward the tissue.

♪ ♪ Sing & Do

After singing your baby's name, inhale

Blow   Wiggle your head forward as you exhale.

Nose   Scrunch your nose.

           Repeat 5 to 10 times.

Baby's Turn:

7. Hold the tissue one or two inches away from the tip of her tiny nose. Make sure you and your baby can still see each other.
8. Ask and encourage your baby to "Blow Nose" as you breathe together. You may notice signs that she is trying to mimic you.

9. Allow a minute for your baby to respond, have patience, and stay there with her until she responds or moves on.

Each time you do this breathing exercise with me I will become more and more involved.

10. Repeat, again asking your baby to "Blow Nose" in your singing voice. And remember, conscious breathing takes repetition to learn.

11. Applaud your baby for effort and move on to the next pose.

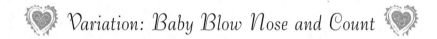

Variation: Baby Blow Nose and Count

Next time you practice Baby Blow, count the breaths aloud. This can be both entertaining and instructive for your baby—while you cultivate inner serenity.

I Love You!
• • • • • • • • • • • • •

(seated version)

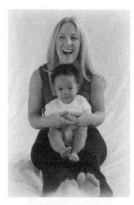

As I get more and more independent, watch our yoga practice shift. As I get a little older and we continue to practice the I Love You! Pose, I may show you how I can originate and move my own arms through part of the pose. I absolutely love moving and you!

1. Sit comfortably. Invite your baby to sit in your lap with his back to your chest.

2. Hold your index fingers out in front of your baby's hands. Invite and help him to grasp your index fingers.

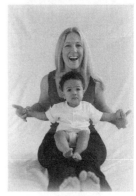

 Sing & Do

| | Assist baby's hands to his heart.
Love . Assist baby's hands and arms in stretching out to the sides.
You! Assist baby's hands and arms into a self-hug and wiggle him from side to side.
Repeat 3 to 5 times.

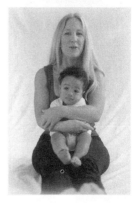

Foreign Language Enhancement

Repeat the I Love You! Pose in any of these foreign languages.
Try Spanish   Te amo!
Try French   Je t'aime! (with a long emphasis on t'aime)
Try Italian   Ti amo!

Can you share the words I Love You in another language that is special to your family?

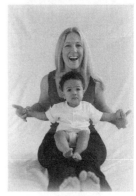

A Magic Pose

Tada

· · · · ·

(Tada is the sanskrit word for Mountain)

 Now that I am crawling I wholeheartedly go after the things that I want. When you help me stand in Tada you move me through space, helping me feel a sense of depth and distance.

1. Sit comfortably, and hold your baby facing you, in a standing position.

2. Support your baby in standing by wrapping your hands under her armpits and around her torso.

3. Let her feet touch and be stimulated by the surface beneath her.

4. Use short punchy sounds and movements to make Tada a success!

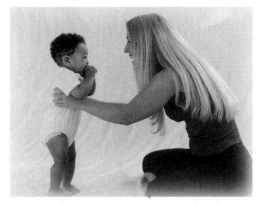

♪ ♪ Sing & Do

Ta	Stand your baby an arm's length away.
Da	Jump baby in toward you.
Ta	Jump her an arm's length away from you.
	Repeat 3 to 5 times.

5. Finish by letting your baby land in your arms and bring her close to your heart.

Ring Around the Yogi

(crawlers version)

 This is another Itsy Bitsy Yoga song that I love to Sing & Do! The first time you show Ring Around the Yogi to me I may be trying to figure out what is going on. So please stick with it. I am just starting to catch on.

1. Decide on the best position for you and your baby in this moment.

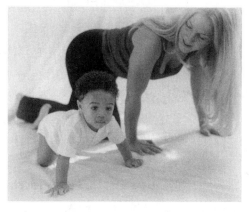

If baby wants to be in your arms:

- Hold your baby in a Diaper Seat Hold (see page 31) and pretend that you're walking like a dinosaur with big, heavy feet as you continue.

If Baby wants to be on the loose:

- Let your baby loose. Come onto your hands and knees, encouraging him to crawl in circles with you.

2. Playfully move in circles as you sing my Ring Around the Yogi song.

♪ Sing & Do

Ring around the yogi
Namaste my friends.
Inhale, exhale,
We all feel grand!
Love is in our hearts
And our minds are full of peaceful thoughts.
Om, delightful om,
Life is fun!

Upside-Down Yogi

 If I love Headstand and Hop Along Yogi, then this will be amazing for us to do together. One reason this pose makes me laugh is that I can see you while my whole body is being bounced! Upside-Down Yogi gives my body the stimulation it needs for healthy physical and emotional development.

1. Sit with your legs extended together and in front of you. Allow the insides of your legs to touch. (This is great pose to do in front of a mirror.)

2. Gently place your baby's back against your shins with her head by your feet. Your baby's spine should rest between your legs.

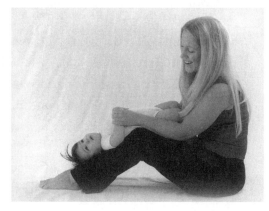

3. Check to see that there is a gap of a few inches between your baby's head and your ankles. If you need to create a gap, slide your baby's feet toward you.

4. Firmly place your hands on the front of your baby's hips. This will keep her safely in place.

5. By bending your knees, slowly elevate your baby up to a 45-degree angle from the floor. If you notice your baby becoming uncomfortable, bring her out of the pose immediately.

6. As your baby remains in place, lengthen your legs and begin to bounce her by bending and lifting your knees up and down while keeping your heels and hips firmly on the floor.

Sing & Do

Upside-down yogi	Bounce legs in a slow to medium pace.
Upside-down yogi	Bounce legs in a slow to medium pace.
Upside-down yogi	Bounce legs in a slow to medium pace.
Real, real SLOW!	Bounce legs in a slow to medium pace.
Upside-down yogi	Bounce legs in a medium to fast pace.
Upside-down yogi	Bounce legs in a medium to fast pace.
Upside-down yogi	Bounce legs in a medium to fast pace.
Read, real FAST!	Bounce legs in a medium to fast pace.
Upside-down yogi	Bounce legs in a fast pace.
Upside-down yogi	Bounce legs in a fast pace.
Upside-down yogi	Bounce legs in a fast pace.
Here we GO!	Bring knees up and baby into a headstand for up to 20 seconds.

7. Straighten your legs back down to the floor and let your baby rest on her back for one minute.

8. Share Heart-Warm Touch with your baby.

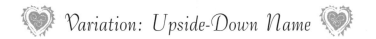

Variation: Upside-Down Name

In the Sing & Do, replace the word yogi with your baby's name and repeat. For instance,

Upside-down Kelly
Upside-down Kelly
Upside-down Kelly
Real, real slow.

Dandasana

· · · · · · · · · · · ·

Do you remember how long it took for me to master sitting and how ready we both were for me to sit? Through the experience of learning how to sit I also learn about the seated staff pose in yoga called Dandasana. Sitting requires my body to engage in a state of stillness, yet remain active in many ways. Maybe that is why it took me so long to master sitting.

1. Sit with your legs extended out in front of you.

2. With your ankles about 12 inches apart, sit your baby between the insides of your knees and facing you.

3. Help straighten his legs and extend them toward you. If he needs a little bit more leg room, reach forward and scoot your baby farther out.

4. Focus on your posture, see what you can learn from your baby as he sits so tall and perfect!

5. Hold your baby's hands as you row through Sing & Do.

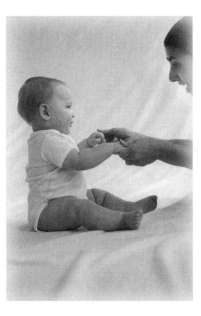

 Sing & Do

Row, row, row with me

Gently up the stream

Verily you're the cutest baby

I have ever seen!

You lean back, baby comes forward.

You lean forward, baby goes back.

You lean back, baby comes forward.

You lean forward, baby goes back.

6. Ask your baby if he'd like to do it again and watch for his response. If he seems to indicate yes, repeat once or twice more.

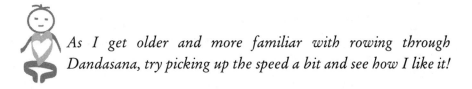

As I get older and more familiar with rowing through Dandasana, try picking up the speed a bit and see how I like it!

7. When you're finished, cheer and give your baby a hug and positive feedback.

So Big
• • • • • • • • •

 When babies do So Big, they are doing yoga's intense west stretch or intense back stretch known as Paschimottānāsana. This pose energizes a baby's spine and improves digestion.

1. Sit on the floor with your legs extended in front of you.

Show Baby How:

2. Invite your baby to face you and sit in between your knees. You can use one small toy to captivate her here.

Sing & Do

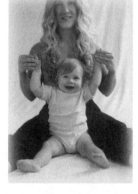

So	(long o) Simultaneously bring both of your hands overhead.
Big	Lean forward from the waist, reaching your arms and torso toward your baby and feet. Repeat one to three times.

3. Let your baby knows that it's her turn.

Baby's Turn, level 1:

5. Try to make eye contact as your baby is sitting between your knees and facing you.

Sing & Do

So	(long o) Hold your baby's hands and lift her arms up as high as she'd like them to go.
Big	Help her quickly bring her hands down toward her feet. Repeat 1 to 5 times.

Baby's Turn, Level 2:

As your baby gets older, move away from her, letting her perform So Big independently. Allow your baby ample time to mimic you. For instance, after you perform So Big five or ten times, she may be about ready to show you her first one. After she's done the pose, mirror it back to her.

Toes to the Nose

● ● ● ● ● ● ● ● ● ● ● ● ● ● ● ● ● ●

(seated, level 2)

Am I a boy or a girl? I ask because hip flexibility in boys is different from that of girls. If I'm a boy, I'm a little less flexible than a girl because of the way my femurs, or leg bones, are positioned into my pelvis.

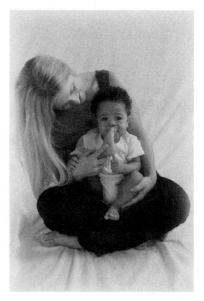

1. Sit your baby in your lap with his back closest to you.

2. If your baby is wearing socks or shoes, take them off.

3. Place your left hand across your baby's belly.

4. Use your right hand to hold your baby's right leg near his ankle. Your thumb rests on his shin and your first few fingers support the back of his leg.

♪ ♪ Sing & Do

Toes	Hold baby's right foot with your right hand.
to the	Bring baby's toes to his nose.
Nose	Tickle his nose with his toes.
	Repeat 3 to 5 times.

Please notice where my flexibility lessens so that we work together in yoga and in life. I know that you don't want to force any of my limbs and that you respect my wishes and body. If I begin to resist the movement, move on to the next pose. Remember, this posture will be here for us to practice again tomorrow.

5. To switch sides, place your right hand on your baby's chest and use your left hand to hold his left leg just above his ankle.

Sing & Do

Toes	Hold baby's foot with your left hand.
to the	Bring baby's toes to his nose.
Nose	Tickle his nose with his toes.
	Repeat 3 to 5 times.

Moon Toe

Moon Toe is called Foot Near Ear, or Akarna Dhanuarāsana, when big people do it in yoga class. After all the crawling I do, it feels so good when my legs stretch into Moon Toe. This pose can also help me go poop when I am having trouble doing so.

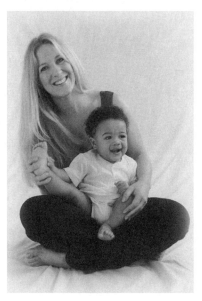

1. Sit comfortably with your baby in your lap facing away from you.

2. Help your baby grab her left foot with her left hand. Use your left hand to reach around your baby's left side and bring her left hand and foot together.

3. Guide your baby in extending her left hand and foot until her leg is at a 45-degree angle from sitting.

4. Follow your baby's cue for when she's ready to bring her left foot back to resting (anywhere from 3 to 5 seconds is good).

Sing & Do

Moon	Baby extends one foot away from her body.
Toe	Baby brings her foot back down and continues to hold it.
	Repeat 3 to 5 times and assist as necessary.

5. To switch sides, use your right hand to help your baby's other hand and foot come together. Repeat using the Sing & Do Technique.

6. Wrap your arms around your baby, slide your hands down her legs, and give her a great big hug!

Yogi Yogi

• • • • • • • • • •

Now that I am crawling, the right and the left sides of my body and brain are integrating with each other. Yogi Yogi is the Itsy Bitsy Yoga version of the Hokey Pokey. I like hearing you sing this song to me. After we do it a few times, you can sing the words to me while we are driving in the car to make me happy then, too!

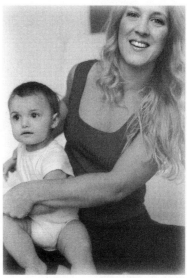

1. If a mirror is nearby, it is wonderful to do Yogi Yogi in front of the mirror.

2. Sit comfortably with your baby in your lap, her back to your chest.

3. Hold your baby's left hand as you begin the Sing & Do.

 ## Sing & Do

You put your left hand in.
Bring baby's left hand away from her body.

You put your left hand out.
Move baby's left hand back by her side.

You put your left hand in.
Bring baby's left hand away from her body.

And circle it about.
Wiggle baby's left hand actively.

You do the Yogi Yogi
Hold both of your baby's hands up toward the ceiling, and move them up and down.

And you turn yourself around.
Hold baby's hands and twist her from side to side by bringing each of her hands to touch the opposite knee.

That's what it's all about!
Giggle, clap, or otherwise communicate that this dance is fun to your baby.

2. Repeat Yogi Yogi using your baby's right hand.

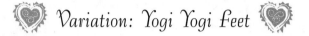 *Variation: Yogi Yogi Feet*

Try Yogi Yogi using feet instead of hands.

Nabhi

• • • • • • •

(Nabhi is the Sanskrit word for wheel)

 Nabhi engages both sides of my brain and body as my arms circle each other. Isn't it amazing how much I am starting to become more like a little toddler than a newborn baby? I feel good about how healthy and strong yet calm I am in my mind and body.

1. Sit comfortably with your baby sitting in your lap or across from you.

2. Hold your hands around his forearms.

3. In an excited and exaggerated fashion say, "Let's do Nabhi!"

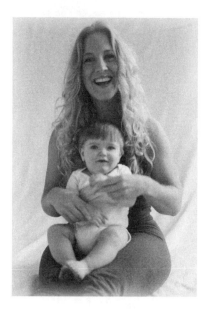

Sing & Do

Nabhi   Churn your baby's hands around each other.

Nabhi   Each repetition of Nabhi marks one complete churn of your baby's hands. Repeat 3 to 8 times.

Baby's Turn

4. As you continue your practice of yoga and Nabhi Pose, allow your baby to take the lead in circling his arms, gradually giving him more and more independence.

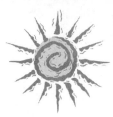

Good Morning Series

·····································

Crawlers

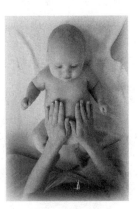

Heart-Warm Touch
page 70

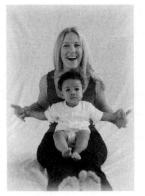

I Love You!
page 155

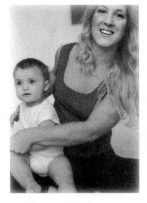

Yogi Yogi
page 167

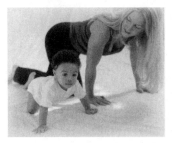

Ring Around the Yogi
page 157

Developmental Play Series

• •

Crawlers

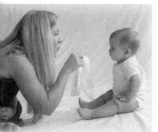

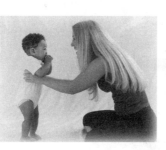

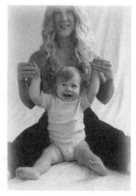

Baby Blow
page 153

Tada
page 156

Dandasana
page 160

So Big
page 162

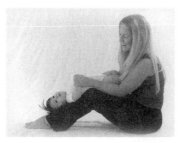

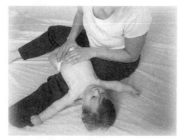

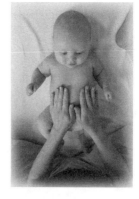

Upside-Down Yogi
page 158

Guppy
page 133

Heart-Warm Touch
page 70

Happy Baby Series

Crawlers

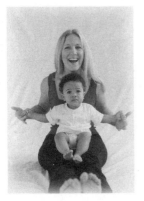

I Love You!
page 155

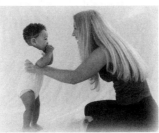
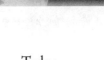

Tada
page 156

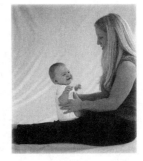

Hop Along Yogi
page 128

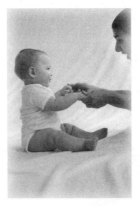

Dandasana
page 160

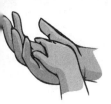

Daddy Series

* * * * * * * * * * * * * *

Crawlers

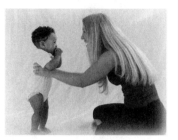

Tada
page 156

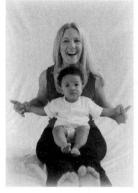

I Love You!
page 155

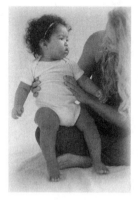

Lampa Season
page 123

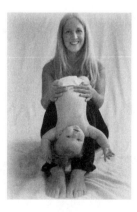

Headstand
page 106

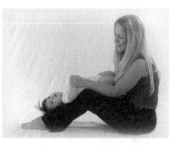

Upside-Down Yogi
page 158

Sleep Well Series

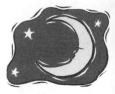

Crawlers

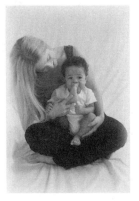

Toes to the Nose
page 164

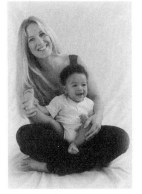

Moon Toe
page 166

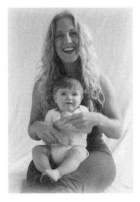

Nabhi
page 169

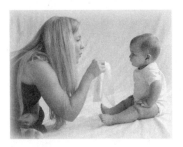

Baby Blow
page 153

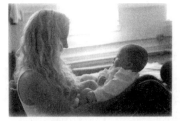

Name Singing
page 101

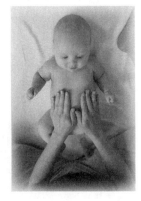

Heart-Warm Touch
page 70

Chapter 10

Yoga for the Almost Walking

When I pull myself up into standing without help, cruise the furniture, squat, or stand on my own I am an Almost-Walking Baby!

As babies near the developmental milestone of walking they pull themselves up into standing on their own, and they begin cruising. Cruising refers to a baby walking sideways while holding onto a piece of furniture with two hands. It typically takes place after the baby has mastered crawling. If your baby begins to cruise the furniture before she crawls, try to put your baby on her tummy more often and let her play on a clean carpeted or blanket-covered floor. Many movement therapists and medical professionals realize the importance crawling before walking so that the child can synchronize the right and the left sides of her body and brain. One innovative mother was so determined for her second child to crawl that she took all the furniture out of the room so her baby had no choice but to be on the floor and crawling.

The almost-walking baby also learns to squat. Squatting helps a baby come in and out of standing and, later, of walking. From a cruising or standing position, a baby may squat for added balance as she holds a small object or toy. Squatting requires a baby's feet to bear weight as the spine lengthens.

Squatting gives babies the sense of being upright as their center of gravity is raised a few inches above the ground. When a baby falls from squatting it is a much shorter distance than when a baby falls from standing. If your baby goes boom, that's what the extra padding in the diaper is for.

As crawling progresses, it may seem that babies are interested in using everything to pull themselves up. Maybe they are, but I don't encourage parents to support their babies in standing. When babies are pulling themselves up and lowering themselves, they are trying to learn how to stand and then return to the floor independently. Sometimes parents misinterpret this, concluding that their baby always wants to stand. Actually, what they want to do is practice coming up and down so they can move onto walking. As a baby practices her up and down transitions, avoid picking her up. If she crawls up onto you, take a moment to lead her lower body back down to the floor in a way that most mirrors her natural way of transitioning when she is leaning against something other than you. By doing this you are helping your baby explore each stage of being an almost-walking baby.

Parents who place crawling babies in walker-seats thinking that their baby will walk sooner are sadly mistaken. Physical therapists agree that walker-seats impede a child's ability to begin walking on time. Walkers give babies a false sense of their center of gravity, and many models don't allow the baby to see his own feet as he moves because of the tray in the front. If you have a walker for your baby, please consider returning it or putting it aside. You'll be glad you did.

As your tot gains independence it is nice to revisit poses you practiced together earlier on. Your baby may recall these poses through the Sing & Do Technique and become a more active yoga participant. Abbey was ten months old and home with mom Beth when mom noticed Abbey's hands up in the air in the "So" part of So Big. Abbey was smiling. Beth thought, "Is Abbey doing So Big?" On an intuitive whim Beth sang out "big!" and Abbey's hands immediately came down toward her feet. Beth realized that Abbey was in fact doing So Big, and she was just as pleased as Abbey was.

Begin to notice how your baby communicates with you during yoga. When Abbey had her hands in the air doing So Big, she was waiting for her mom to follow through and say "big." That was Abbey's cue to flop her arms down. Abbey was communicating through movement. Although your baby may not speak to you in words at this time, you are establishing lines of communication for respect and a clear-spoken child later in life.

As you practice yoga with your baby, leave an empty thirty to sixty seconds between poses so that you can let him finish what you started with him, or communicate with you. Remember to practice what I call "Baby Pace" with your tot (see page 147). Slow down and allow ample time between poses so you will be aware of the yoga poses your baby is showing you. As you and your tot become familiar with the poses, you'll notice your baby giving you preverbal cues (with body language) as to what pose would work best in this moment. It's up to you to watch and listen.

In this chapter, your baby will learn plenty of interactive yoga poses that specifically help with balance and moving through space—two vital precursors to walking. The way your baby approaches her yoga will differ, depending on what developmental process she is mastering. As movements and poses are repeated, they will flow much more rhythmically for both of you. She'll remember much of what you do now with her for months to come. Your baby now wants to play with you. Have fun!

As you begin the yoga practice for almost walkers:

- Clear the space.
- Gather a handkerchief or lightweight scarf for Te Lol Jah, the Hindi version of peek-a-boo.
- Put any nearby small toys away.
- When necessary, consider demonstrating the pose to your tot using a doll or stuffed animal.
- Find a full-length or decent-sized mirror to help you see your tot's reactions.
- Play soft music.
- Start with Belly Breathing (pages 24–25) and the Heart-Warm Touch (page 70).
- End with any of the relaxation techniques described on pages 34–37.

Twistee

• • • • • • • •

Twistee is a seated spinal twist designed just for me! It tones my belly and refreshes my lungs if I have respiratory problems. As we practice Twistee, invite me to gain more and more independence by letting my fingers wrap around your index finger or thumb. Eventually I will be the one leading us both into the twist.

1. While sitting in a comfortable cross-legged position, place your baby in your lap with her back to your chest.

2. Wrap your arms around her and lovingly hold her hands with yours.

3. Guide her right hand to her left knee, then her left hand to her right knee.

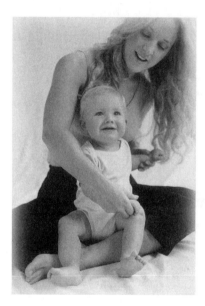

Sing & Do

Twist	Bring right hand to her left knee.
Tee	Bring left hand to her right knee.
	Repeat 6 to 8 times.

4. Let your baby know how much fun you are having with her!

Half Moon

In Half Moon, one half of my belly compresses while and the other side is extended, helping my belly feel good. As we rest in Half Moon Pose, you'll notice me smile because of the way you and yoga make me feel.

Show Baby How:

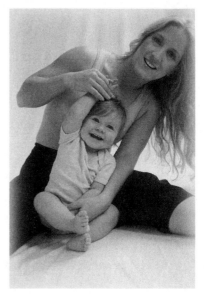

1. With your baby crawling freely around you, sit comfortably with your legs crossed.

2. On an inhalation, lift your right arm up overhead with your palm facing you. Exhale as you drop your shoulder down.

3. With your next exhale, tilt your body to your left side.

4. While in the pose, call your baby and ask, "Half Moon, do you want to try?" (It helps to sing the pose name, Half Moon, as you ask.)

5. Take several breaths as you sing "Half Moon" and relax further into the pose.

6. On an inhalation, slowly return to upright. Exhale as you let your arm float down to your side. Switch sides, extending your left arm overhead and tilting to your right side.

Baby's Turn:

7. Let your baby know it's his turn and sit him in your lap with his back against your chest.

8. Place your left hand over your baby's belly while using your right hand to hold his right hand.

9. With your right hand, lift your baby's hand up and over his shoulder.

10. While you both remain seated firmly on the floor, completely tilt both of you over to your left side by bending at the waist.

13. Rest to the side for 5 to 10 seconds as you sing "Half Moon" and your baby settles into this pose.

14. Slowly lift yourselves to the upright position.

15. Switch sides and repeat one to three times using my Sing & Do technique.

Sing & Do

Up	Your right hand on baby's belly. Left hand holds baby's left hand and arm up.
Up	Tilt you and your baby to the right by bending at your waist.
Away	Remain in this side bend for 5 to 10 seconds.
Half Moon	Inhale and float back to upright. Alternate sides and repeat.

16. Thank your baby for his participation.

Jumping Bean

Jumping Bean makes me cheerful as my feet lightly touch the earth and my heart reaches for the sky! Since I am an almost-walking baby I am set on learning how to move up and down while standing. And, that's what you do with me in Jumping Bean.

1. Kneel or stand on your knees and place a pillow under your knees for comfort.

2. With your baby facing you, support her in a standing position by holding her under her armpits.

3. Hop your baby so she is 6 to 8 inches or a comfortable distance in front of you.

4. During the Sing & Do, use a high-energy voice to sing "Jumping, jumping, jumping bean!" to match this high-energy pose.

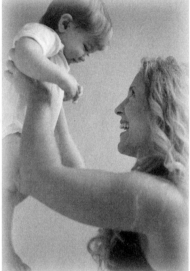

Sing & Do

Jump-	Lift baby up.
ing	Baby's feet touch floor.
Jump-	Lift baby up.
ing	Baby's feet touch floor.
Jump-	Lift baby up.
ing	Baby's feet touch floor.
Bean!!	With baby standing, wiggle her from side to side.
	Repeat 1 to 3 times.

6. Good job! I know Jumping Bean is a workout for you, too. Bring your baby in close for a hug.

Standing Knee to Chest

 Standing Knee to Chest improves my digestion and lets me play with my balance as I learn to stand. I like to think of Standing Knee to Chest as a more grown-up version of Apana Pose.

1. Sit with your legs extended in front of you in a V shape.

2. Rest your baby's back against your chest as you support him in standing.

3. Position your left hand over your baby's belly. Your right hand can hold his nearest shin, just below his knee.

Sing & Do

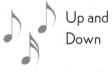

Knee	Bring baby's knee up and toward his chest.
Up and	Hold for 1 to 5 seconds.
Down	Lower your hand and baby's foot to floor. Repeat 1 to 5 times with each leg.

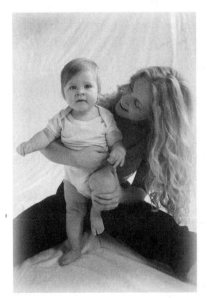

Sitting Tree

Sitting Tree is found in grown-up yoga practices as Head to Knee Pose, or Jānu Sīrsāsana. Sitting Tree is another great pose one for my digestion and also helps to activate and tone my kidneys, which helps keep me pure, as every baby should be!

Show Baby How:

1. With your baby nearby, sit with your legs extended in front of you. Bring one heel in to touch the side of your thigh or lower leg, whatever is more comfortable for you.

2. Take a deep breath as you raise both hands above your head. Sing the word "sitting."

3. Exhale as you bring your hands down toward your extended foot and sing "tree."

4. Repeat steps 1 through 3 with your other leg extended.

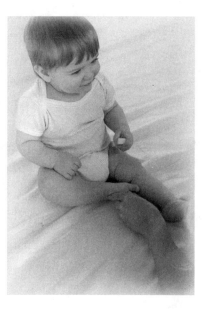

Baby's Turn:

5. Spread your knees apart enough to snuggle your baby as she sits facing you.

6. Help your baby straighten her legs toward you. If her legs need a little bit more room, reach forward and scoot your baby toward your feet.

7. Tuck one of your baby's ankles into the side of her other thigh.

Sing & Do

Sitting   Help her lift her hands overhead.

Tree   Help her lower her hands over her extended leg toward her toes.

Repeat 3 to 5 times before switching legs.

8. Clap together and praise your baby.

Shoulderstand

· · · · · · · · · · · · · ·

With your help I can go up into Shoulderstand easily, safely, and for many good reasons. Shoulderstand helps grown-ups and babies alike alleviate asthma and throat and urinary problems, and helps with digestion and elimination. Also, in Shoulderstand my brain and glands receive a fresh supply of oxygen-rich blood.

1. Place your baby on his back on the carpet or blanket.

2. At your baby's feet, kneel atop a pillow.

3. Grasp his thighs and hold firmly as you prepare for this inverted posture.

4. As you perform Shoulderstand with your baby, keep his head, neck, and shoulders in contact with the floor.

5. Slowly lift his legs upward and toward his chest, until his thighs are over his chest.

6. Hold for 8 to 25 seconds or until your baby signals that he's ready to come out of the pose by turning his head or arching his back.

7. Lower your baby's legs and pause.

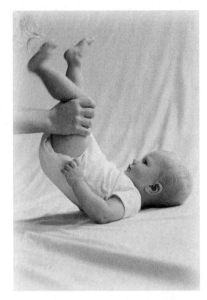

♪ ♪ Sing & Do

Shoulder   Lift legs up.

Stand   Hold for 8 to 25 seconds. Lower baby's legs.

              Repeat 1 to 3 times.

Fish

· · · · ·

Like Guppy Pose, Fish Pose expands my chest and lungs while stretching my neck and upper and middle back. With this pose my glands receive blood and oxygen to help them work well and keep me healthy!

1. With your baby lying on her back, kneel or sit on your baby's left side facing her belly.

2. Slide your right hand with palm facing up and under her upper to mid back. We will be creating a slight arch in your baby's mid-back, lifting her heart.

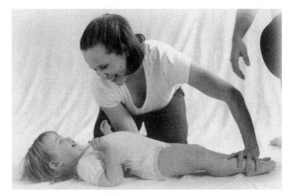

3. Gently hold your baby's feet with your left hand.

In Fish Pose my head, tush, and legs remain on the floor and my heart opens to you.

4. With your right hand, lift your baby's back off the floor slightly, allowing her back to arch lightly.

5. Using a sweet voice, it's Sing & Do time, but this time it's more like sing and hold.

Sing & Do

Nice Job   Continue supporting her in Fish Pose for 5 to 15 seconds.
Fish Pose
You're doing
Fish Pose   Start to bring baby out of Fish Pose as in step 6 below.

6. Slowly lower your right hand and baby's mid-back to the floor. Remove
   your hands and let your baby come back into sitting.

Hindi Peek-a-Boo

• • • • • • • • • • • • • • • • • • •

(Te lol jah! means Peek-a-Boo! in Hindi.)

 Babies all over the world love peek-a-boo. Peek-a-boo teaches us that things are still there even when we don't see them. Let me hide behind a cloth diaper, face cloth, or big ball as we do Hindi Peek-a-Boo.

Show Baby How:

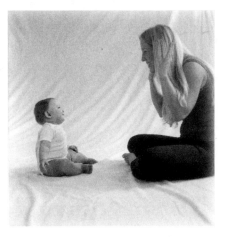

1. Sit comfortably with your baby nearby and facing you.

 ### Sing & Do

Te lol	Cover your eyes.
Jah !	Uncover your eyes.
	Repeat until you have his interest.

Baby's Turn, Stage 1:

2. Sit with your legs extended in front of you. Seat your baby between your knees facing you.

3. Position your hands two inches in front of your baby's eyes.

 ### Sing & Do

Te lol	Lightly cover your baby's eyes.
Jah !	Uncover your baby's eyes.
	Repeat 3 to 5 times.

Baby's Turn, Stage 2:

4. In stage 2 of Te lol Jah both you and your baby will cover your eyes independently.

Sing & Do

Te lol   You cover your eyes. Baby covers his eyes.

Jah!   You uncover your eyes. Baby uncovers his eyes.

Slowly and playfully repeat several times.

5. When given some time, your baby will mimic you and play along. When you see him doing any portion of the pose, applaud enthusiastically. Your baby loves to please you!

Clappy Happy Namaste

 When I clap my hands, I do so happily in front of my heart. As I feel my hands touching each other I am experiencing my own Heart-Warm Touch. If I am still learning about clapping my hands together, Clappy Happy Namaste is good practice.

Show Baby How:

1. Sit comfortably with your baby nearby.

2. Cheerfully perform the Clappy Happy Namaste Sing & Do with a high level of excitement.

 ## Sing & Do

Clappy	Continuously clap your hands.
Happy	
Namaste	
	Repeat until you have baby's attention.

Baby's Turn, Stage 1:

 ## Sing & Do

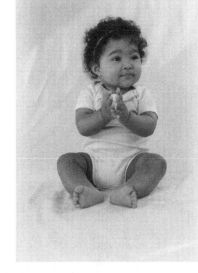

Clappy	Help baby clap her hands together.
Happy	
Namaste	
	Repeat 3 to 5 times.

Baby's Turn, Stage 2:

3. Give your baby a moment or two to explore clapping her hands together as you sing Clappy Happy Namaste more slowly than before. Repeat as necessary.

Candle Breathing

Candle Breathing allows you the opportunity to come into my world and see how I learn things. By watching me mindfully you become part of all the little magical moments that lead up to me doing what you show me or what I am trying to accomplish on my own!

1. If you have an unlit number birthday candle or an unlit votive candle in your home, it will be a useful tool in this breathing exercise.

2. Sit comfortably facing your baby.

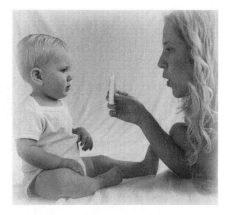

Show Baby How:

3. Hold the unlit candle just below your chin.

4. Momentarily close your eyes as you take a deep long breath in.

5. Open your eyes and make eye contact with him as you loosely pucker your lips.

6. Repeat the phrase "blow the candle" and exhale, pretending that you are blowing out the unlit candle. Repeat several times.

Baby's Turn:

7. Hold the candle for your baby near his mouth.

8. Encourage your baby to "blow the candle," and wait for his response.

9. Explore demonstrating for your baby and allowing him to mimic you.

10. At a time when your baby is becoming more verbal, notice the many subtle lip formations that are necessary for both blowing out a candle and talking.

11. Applaud your baby for his effort.

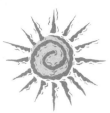

Good Morning Series

· · · · · · · · · · · · · · · · · · · ·

Almost Walkers

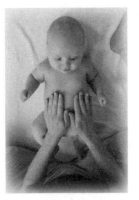

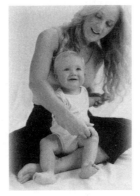

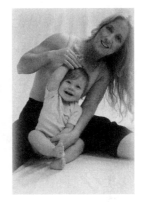

Heart-Warm Touch
page 70

Twistee
page 179

Half Moon
page 180

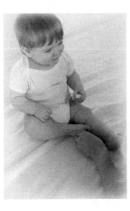

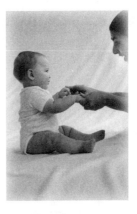

Sitting Tree
page 184

Dandasana
page 160

Developmental Play Series

Almost Walkers

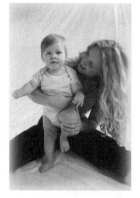

Standing Knee to Chest
page 183

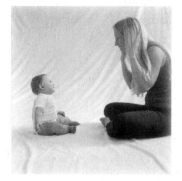

Hindi Peek-a-Boo
page 189

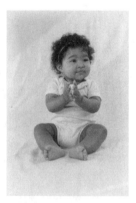

Clappy Happy Namaste
page 191

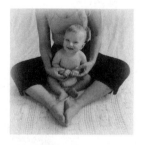

Butterfly
page 125

Happy Baby Series

· ·

Almost Walkers

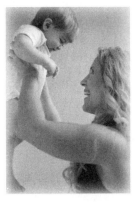

Jumping Bean
page 182

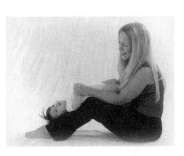

Upside-Down Yogi
page 158

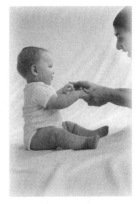

Dandasana
page 160

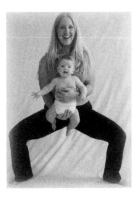

Divine Drops
page 79

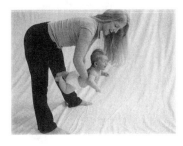

Womb Wings
page 81

Daddy Series

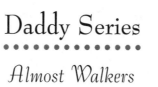

Almost Walkers

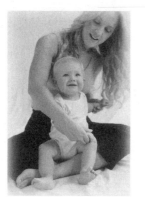

Twistee
page 179

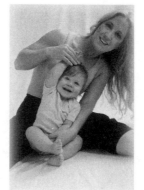

Half Moon
page 180

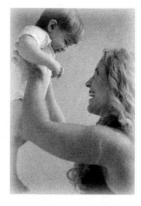

Jumping Bean
page 182

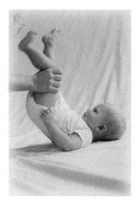

Shoulderstand
page 186

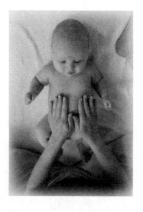

Heart-Warm Touch
page 70

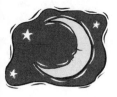

Sleep Well Series

Almost Walkers

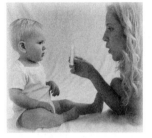

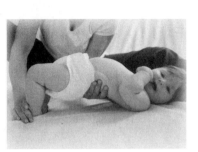

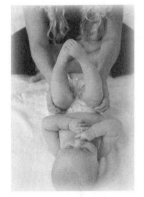

Candle Breathing
page 192

Bridge
page 104

Apana
page 72

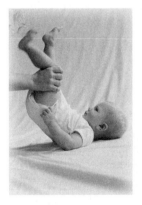

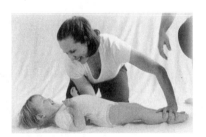

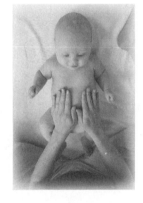

Shoulderstand
page 186

Fish
page 187

Heart-Warm Touch
page 70

Chapter 11

Yoga for Walkers

 My parents made a big deal when I walked across the room completely on my own. I have to admit, I was proud too. It felt so good to stand tall and walk like big people do.

When babies first learn how to walk, they do not move forward in a straight line. They walk in a roundabout fashion. Perhaps this is why some early walkers resort to crawling toward something they want to get to in a hurry. In this chapter you will learn that a walking tot's yoga practice can be as active as he is.

The 3 Keys

What makes a walking tot's yoga practice successful? The three key actions are:

1. **Move** in and out of the practice.
2. **Show** a baby the pose.
3. **See** a baby's movement initiations and desires.

Key #1 MOVE: Move In and Out of the Practice.

As you share yoga with a mobile tot, the entire room is the yoga mat. Walking tots can explore the room freely during yoga. A mobile baby's movement should not be strictly confined unless it's to protect him from injury. After yoga class, Mom Beth was frustrated because Ethan, her sixteen-month-old son, would not sit with her and do a series of yoga poses like the other one-year-olds in class who had been practicing yoga for weeks or months longer. Ethan was all over the place. He explored the studio, the other babies, and me. I could see his mother's frustration, but I knew exploring would lead Ethan to comfort and his desire to experience yoga. During Ethan's second class, he'd do one or two poses, then wander off and return again for another pose or more of the one he had just done. Practicing yoga poses like adults, consecutively and in one sitting, will eventually take place, especially if a baby starts yoga before he is mobile.

Key #2 SHOW: Show a Baby the Pose.

You've done a great job facilitating your baby's yoga during the first year of his life. Now more than ever before, your animation when demonstrating the poses becomes key. Since your baby is more independent and capable of initiating and mimicking yoga poses, you want to provide clear instruction with your body. In addition to demonstrating a yoga pose, you can put a doll or stuffed animal into the yoga pose you are practicing. When you let your baby preview a yoga pose, he feels respected and knows what is asked. He will involve himself intellectually and physically as he studies your movements.

Let your demonstration of a pose be a visual and auditory experience for a baby. As you show a yoga pose, sing the pose's name and follow my Sing & Do Technique. Typically, when you ask a baby, "Where's your feet?" the baby will grab her feet. Well, the same applies in yoga. When you sing "Tree Pose," the baby who practices yoga regularly will do Tree Pose. Yoga gives babies a sense of achievement.

When you show a baby a pose you open the channel of communication for them to show you a pose too! Perhaps your baby will show her interest by initiating a component of the pose. For instance, if a baby sits in my lap and bounces, that may be her way of asking me to do Hop Along Yogi with her. Notice where your baby's interests lie in this moment and move from there. This brings us to Key #3, *See*.

Key #3 SEE: See a Baby's Movement Initiations and Desires.

The pose Ethan started to do did not coincide with the pose I was teaching at the time. For Ethan it was very important that we supported him in doing the pose he wanted to do. One of the most valuable lessons parents learn in tots' yoga classes is how to observe what their baby wants to do and let that lead the practice, rather than follow a specific agenda. This doesn't mean that we let babies in class quit practicing yoga to play with a ball. It means that we include the ball in the practice and we continue practicing yoga.

Discover what pose your baby is interested in by observing his body position and movements. For example, one of Ethan's starting poses was Lampa, and we knew he wanted to do Lampa when both feet were firmly on the floor and he was bending his knees. Learn the poses that your baby wants to do first, and then you can move through the others.

Sometimes, it comes down to timing. Olivia, Stacy's seventeen-month-old daughter, seems to enjoy yoga but her mom felt Olivia was always a pose or two behind her class. You see, Olivia was learning yoga in Baby Pace. As I explained earlier (page 147), Baby Pace gives babies and toddlers the extra time needed to process and act upon what we are showing, singing, or asking them. By coming to class, Olivia saw how Baby Pace worked by watching the others temporally suspend the boundedness of time and the feeling of "we must do this right now." In yoga, parents slow down and see their baby's intention clearly.

As you begin the yoga practice for walkers:

- Clear the space.
- Gather a flower, sachet, or any handheld object in your home that has a pleasant odor for Flower Breathing.
- Put any nearby small toys away.
- When necessary, demonstrate the pose to your tot using a doll or stuffed animal.
- Play soft music.
- Start with Belly Breathing (pages 24–25) and the Heart-Warm Touch (page 70).
- End with any of relaxation techniques described on pages 34–37.

Flower Breathing

 Breathing gives me life, but with practice and focus it can also give me a peaceful, calm feeling that will be great for me to learn before I turn two. Watch my throat, heart, and belly rise up toward the sky as I inhale with my nose. In flower breathing, I'll first get to watch your throat, heart, and belly rise and then I'll try to mimic you!

1. Have a flower, sachet, or any handheld object in your home that smells good nearby. (An artificial flower topped with a drop of essential oil works well.)

2. Face your baby and sit comfortably.

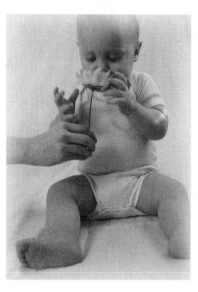

Show Baby How:

3. Hold the flower or scented object a little below your nose.

4. Make eye contact with her.

5. Inhale as you pretend to smell the sweetest smell you have ever smelled. Let the deep inhalation fill your belly and heart.

6. Exhale completely with a satisfied *mmm* sound.

7. Repeat, demonstrating for her one to three times.

Baby's Turn:

8. Hold the flower or scent-filled object to your baby's nose.

Remember, your animation and interest in breathing stimulates me to mimic you!

9. Encourage her to "smell" as you inhale vivaciously and exhale satisfied, using the Sing & Do Technique.

Sing & Do

(Baby's name) smell?	Invite baby to smell the flower.
Smell for Mommy (Daddy, etc.).	Hold flower for baby to smell.
Let's smell together.	Both you and baby smell flower.

Continue with your baby for as long as she is interested.

10. Affirm "good smelling" to your baby.

Lampa

· · · · · · ·

(Lampa is the Sanskrit word for jump)

 In Lampa Pose my standing body will learn how to jump up and down. As you show me Lampa, watch my body slowly work toward doing it. Jumping is an amazing full-body movement and involves everything from head to toe, so allow me lots of time to figure it out as we practice yoga!

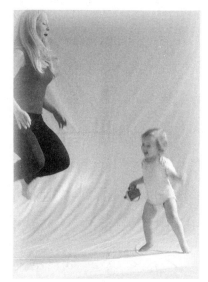

Show Baby How:

1. Near but independent of your baby, begin to jump up and down singing "Lampa!"

Baby's Turn, Stage 1:

2. Using a pillow under your knees, come into kneel-standing.

3. With your baby standing in front of you, place your hands under his armpits.

Sing & Do

Lam-	Baby stands as you lift him 3 to 12 inches off the floor.
pa	Lower baby's feet to the floor. Repeat 1 to 3 times.

Baby's Turn, Stage 2:

4. Stand in front of your baby as he stands, too.

5. Exclaim "Lampa, Lampa, Lampa" as you begin to jump up and down. Let your baby try to copy you.

Lampa   Jump up and down independently.

Lampa   Jump up and down independently.

You can do it!   Pause for 20 seconds, letting only your baby begin to jump.

Lampa, Lampa

 In Lampa, you know I am starting to do this pose completely on my own if I start coming down into a semi-squat or having a little bounce in my knees.

6. Thank your baby for doing a good job!

Tree
· · · · ·

With recognition and practice I will bring my foot up into Tree Pose as I hold your hand or something else for balance. I absolutely love doing Tree Pose and watching the reactions of my family or friends. It makes me so happy to have an audience of people who love me and love to see my body move! Tree Pose is good for my self-esteem, balance, leg strength, and coordination.

Show Baby How:

1. With your baby nearby, stand tall and gaze at a nonmoving point.

2. Lift one foot and bring it to the side of your other calf or thigh.

3. Hold for 3 to 10 seconds as you call out *"Look, Tree Pose"* several times.

4. Repeat with the other leg.

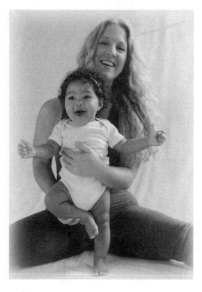

Baby's Turn, Stage 1:

5. Kneel-stand on your pillow or sit behind your standing child.

6. Wrap your left arm around him, placing your left hand on her belly.

7. With your right hand hold her right foot.

8. Ask her to lift the foot you are holding into tree pose.

9. Use a fairylike and enchanted voice as you continue with Sing & Do.

Sing & Do

Tree pose	Lift or guide her in placing the foot you're holding on the inside calf of the leg your baby is standing on.
You're doing it	Hold her foot in place.
Tree Pose	Lower the foot.
Good	(baby's name) Pause and bask in the joy of yoga!
	Repeat 1 to 3 times before switching feet.

Baby's Turn, Stage 2:

I may need to hold a hand or piece of furniture for balance when I do Tree Pose.

10. Stand in front of your child and hold one of her hands.

11. Pick your left foot up and place it in Tree Pose (see step 2).

12. While holding Tree Pose, look at your baby and call out "Tree Pose! Look who's doing Tree Pose, Tree Pose!"

13. Ask your baby to try the pose and encourage her to lift one foot into Tree Pose. If necessary, use one of your hands to help lift your baby's foot into Tree Pose.

14. Tell her what a great job she did as you smile and clap.

Down Dog

Down Dog is something I did when I was learning to crawl and now it's something that I do because I want to. Down Dog is an exhilarating pose for my body: it invigorates my brain and rejuvenates my spirit! It is good for babies who have trouble with asthma or who need to strengthen their muscles.

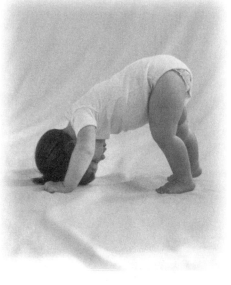

Show Baby How:

1. Bring your hands and knees to the floor. Keep your back flat like a table. Your knees are under your hips and hands under your shoulders.

2. Curl your toes under and lift your hips up. Check to see that your feet are at least hip distance apart.

3. Press into your fingertips and adjust your hands so that you are comfortable.

4. Call your baby over and say "Down Dog. Look, Down Dog!"

Baby's Turn:

5. With your baby standing, kneel-stand behind him and place your hands on the front of his hips.

6. Encourage his hands to reach forward and onto the floor. (A small toy placed on the floor where you hope his hands will go is useful.)

7. If necessary, pull his hips up, making sure that his feet and hands can still touch the floor.

8. Once he's carrying weight on his hands and feet, let go of his waist and hips.

9. Tell him, "Good job. You're doing Down Dog."

10. Clap together with a sense of accomplishment!

Star

The side-stepping motion in Star Pose is similar to cruising, when I side-step to walk along furniture. Since I am now walking, I have integrated cruising into my movement repertoire and can fully enjoy the comfort of Star Pose. This pose begins like yoga's Five-Pointed Star Pose, but then my hands and feet move synchronously, allowing my body awareness and grace to expand exponentially!

1. You can be either fully standing or kneel-standing as you begin Star Pose.

2. Stand your baby in front of you and hold her hands out to the sides so that she makes a star shape.

3. Shift your weight to your left foot, raising your right foot off the floor and perhaps your baby's footing will follow.

4. Return your right foot to the floor which will now give the necessary support to raise the left foot off the floor.

5. Continue rocking from side to side with your baby as you alternate the lifted foot and sing "Twinkle, Twinkle Little Star."

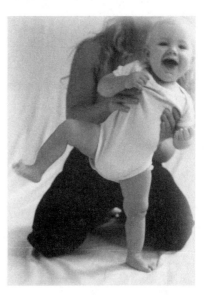

Sing & Do

Twin-	Shift weight to right foot, lift left leg to side.
kle	Shift weight to left foot, lift right leg to side.
Twin-	Shift weight to right foot, lift left leg to side.
kle	Shift weight to left foot, lift right leg to side.
Lit-	Shift weight to right foot, lift left leg to side.
tle	Shift weight to left foot, lift right leg to side.
Star	Shift weight to right foot, lift left leg to side.

How	Shift weight to left foot, lift right leg to side.
I	Shift weight to right foot, lift left leg to side.
Won-	Shift weight to left foot, lift right leg to side.
der	Shift weight to right foot, lift left leg to side.
What	Shift weight to left foot, lift right leg to side.
You	Shift weight to right foot, lift left leg to side.
Are	Shift weight to left foot, lift right leg to side.
Up	Shift weight to right foot, lift left leg to side.
A-	Shift weight to left foot, lift right leg to side.
bove	Shift weight to right foot, lift left leg to side.
The	Shift weight to left foot, lift right leg to side.
World	Shift weight to right foot, lift left leg to side.
So	Shift weight to left foot, lift right leg to side.
High	Shift weight to right foot, lift left leg to side.
Like	Shift weight to left foot, lift right leg to side.
A	Shift weight to right foot, lift left leg to side.
Dia-	Shift weight to left foot, lift right leg to side.
mond	Shift weight to right foot, lift left leg to side.
In	Shift weight to left foot, lift right leg to side.
The	Shift weight to right foot, lift left leg to side.
Sky	Shift weight to left foot, lift right leg to side

8. Since your baby loves repetition, repeat step 5 but this time do Star Pose completely on your own and let your baby take her time as she explores Star Pose completely on her own.

Warrior

· · · · · · · · ·

 The word warrior makes it sound like this would be a scary pose, but it is actually a pose about harmony, poise, power, trust, and balance. It's never too early for me to start leaning about these good traits. When I do Warrior Pose on my own, it can help make my legs strong and tone my abdominal region.

1. Kneel-stand, using a pillow under your knees for extra cushioning or sit.

2. With your baby standing at your right side, place your left hand under his belly.

3. With your left hand still under his belly, lean him forward and place your right hand under his right leg.

4. While baby keeps his left foot on the floor, lift his right leg up and guide him forward until he is parallel with the floor.

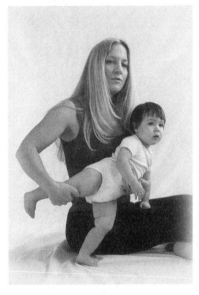

 To help me reach forward with my arms, it's nice to have a coffee table or other little table for me to rest my arms on as my leg lifts.

5. Let him know he is in Warrior Pose by repeating the words "Warrior Pose" several times.

6. Repeat on the other side.

Train

Train helps me work off excessive energy, allowing me to be focused and content. The choo-choo sound that we'll make in Train is a rejuvenating breathing exercise!

1. Stand or sit comfortably with your baby.

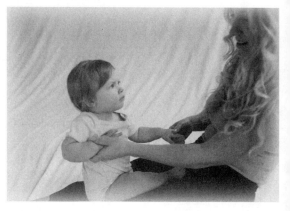

Show Baby How:

2. With your arms at your sides, bend your elbows and extend your hands out in front of you (in a handshake position).

3. Slowly start to pull your right elbow back toward you as your left elbow moves forward.

Sing & Do

Chug   Swing or chug your bent elbows back and forth in an alternating fashion repeatedly.

A-chuga
Choo
Choo

          Continue for 15 to 30 seconds.

Baby's Turn, Stage 1:

4. Kneel or sit across from your standing or sitting baby.

5. Hold both of his hands in your own and assist your baby in chugging his arms back and forth like the wheels on a train.

Sing & Do

Chug	Guide your baby's arms in chugging back-and-forth motion repeatedly.
A-chuga	
Whoo,	(it's a windy sound)
Whoo	Blow out your breath through pursed lips.
	Continue for as long as your baby would like.

6. Give your baby positive encouragement and applause. Feel good about how wonderful it is to teach him yoga!

Baby's Turn, Stage 2:

7. Repeat Train's Sing & Do as your baby explores doing Train independently.

8. Support his efforts by mirroring him and singing Chug A-chuga, Whoo! Whoo!

Half Bow

This pose is especially good for my spine and my belly. Do you know that scoliosis can begin during infancy? It's true; my spine is being formatted by my holding patterns. Yoga is one of the wonderful ways for me to bring my spine into it natural alignment.

1. Entice your baby to lie on her belly in front of you.

2. Sit facing the right side of her body.

3. Hold your baby's right hand with your right hand.

4. Lightly hold your baby's right shin with your left hand.

5. Keeping hold of baby's hand, gently lift her foot up near her tush.

6. Guide her in holding her foot by moving her hand back toward her foot. Ask for her help.

7. If necessary, use your hand to gently clasp her foot and hand together to seal the Half Bow Pose.

8. Sing the pose name "Half Bow" and give your baby positive feedback.

9. Repeat steps 1 through 8 on the other side.

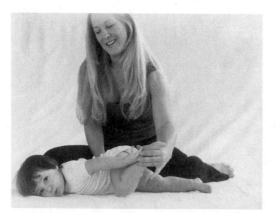

Ring Around the Yogi

Moving in circles of various speeds can be useful in taking the edge off what some call the terrible twos. You may even catch me moving in a circle completely on my own because it is so fun!

1. Stand with your baby and hold hands with him. Begin walking in a circle with your baby.

Sing & Do

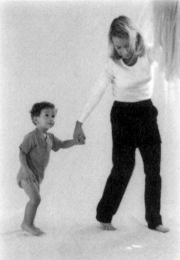

Ring around the Yogi	Hold hands and circle continuously.
Namaste my friends. Inhale, exhale, We all feel grand!	Throw your hands up in the air.

2. Both you and your baby come down to the floor onto your hands and knees, on all fours. (This is Table Pose in yoga, and similar to a crawling position.)

3. Let your movements and sounds encourage your baby to follow along in Sing & Do.

Sing & Do

Love is in our hearts	March hands up and down on floor.
And our minds are full of peaceful thoughts.	Continue marching hands.
Om, delightful Om,	Sit back on your heels and press your palms together in front of your heart.
Life is fun!	Clap hands on your thighs, then playfully throw both hands up overhead!

4. Applaud with your baby, then hug him or do a high five!

5. Repeat once or twice.

Om Mudra

· · · · · · · · · · ·

(*Om* means absolute and *Mudra* means seal in Sanskrit.)

 Om Mudra is part of my natural development and can be compared to the pincher grasp reflex. Notice how good I am at picking up small edible objects like Cheerios. It is my pincher grasp reflex that initially allows me to be so proficient at it.

1. Sit comfortably near your baby.

Show Baby How:

2. Gaze downward or close your eyes. Take a deep breath in and out.

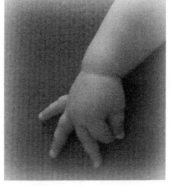

Sing & Do
"Om" is pronounced to rhyme with home.

O   (long & constant) Press index finger and thumb together.

M   (humming sound) Hold index finger and thumb together. Release.

3. Release and repeat several times for your baby's eyes to see and her brain to digest.

Baby's Turn:

4. Help your baby bring her thumb and index finger together. Try letting her feel responsible for the action.

5. Invite your baby to Sing & Do "Om" with you as in step 2.

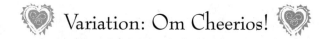 Variation: Om Cheerios!

Babies and toddlers take hold of the world with their hands. Use Cheerios or some kind of finger food to motivate your baby to bring his fingers together into Om Mudra and develop finger dexterity.

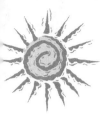

Good Morning Series

· ·

Walkers

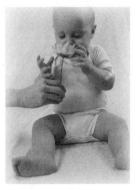

Flower Breathing
page 203

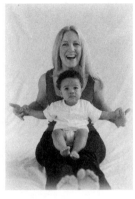

I Love You!
page 155

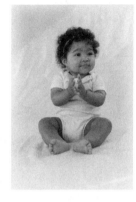

Clappy Happy Namaste
page 191

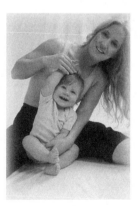

Half Moon
page 180

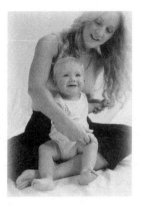

Twistee
page 179

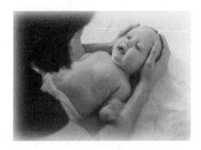

Baby Planet
page 78

Developmental Play Series

Walkers

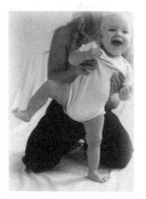

Star
page 211

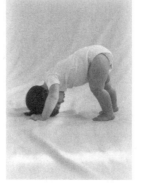

Down Dog
page 209

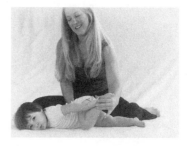

Half Bow
page 216

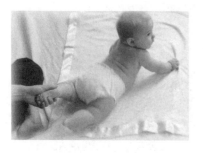

Kicky Cobra
page 132

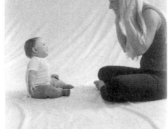

Hindi Peek-a-Boo
page 189

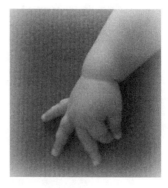

Om Mudra
page 219

Happy Baby Series

* * * * * * * * * * * * * * * * * * * *

Walkers

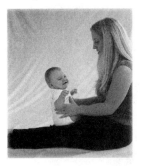

Hop Along Yogi
page 128

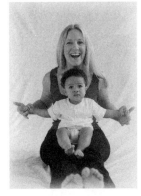

I Love You!
page 155

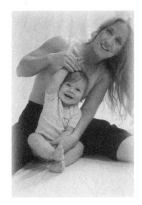

Half Moon
page 180

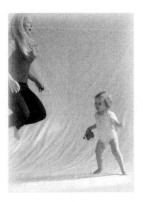

Lampa
page 205

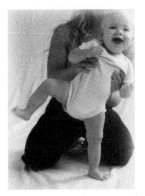

Star
page 211

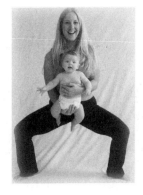

Divine Drops
page 79

Daddy Series

• • • • • • • • • • • • •

Walkers

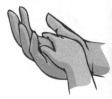

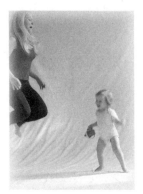

Lampa
page 205

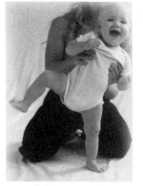

Star
page 211

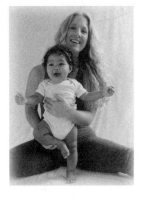

Tree
page 207

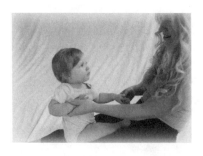

Train
page 214

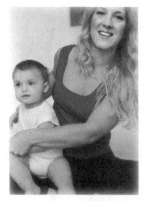

Yogi Yogi
page 167

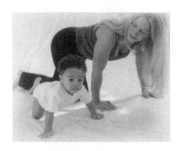

Ring Around the Yogi
page 217

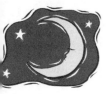

Sleep Well Series

Walkers

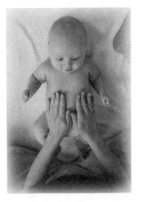

Heart-Warm Touch
page 70

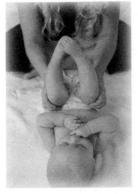

Apana
page 72

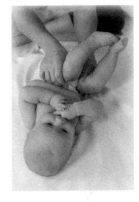

Corkscrew
page 74

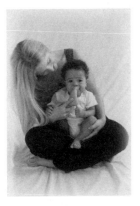

Toes to the Nose
page 164

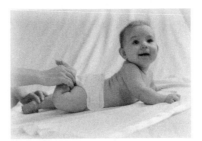

Tushie Touches
page 102

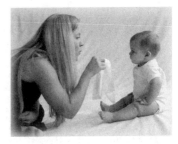

Baby Blow
page 153

Chapter 12

Yoga Through Childhood

 Let's design a customized yoga routine for your growing child! First, record the names of ten of his all-time favorite yoga poses below. Include the page numbers too. We'll need them later. The poses you and your toddler select can come from any chapter (see the appendix as a reference tool).

Pose   Page #

1. _____

2. _____

3. _____

4. _____

5. _____

6. _____

7. _____

8. _____

9. _____

10. _____

Next, we'll set the order of poses for your toddler's customized yoga routine. Reorder the list you made above, putting the poses in order by page number, with the highest page number listed first. This becomes the sequence or flow of your toddler's yoga routine.

Pose   Page # *(highest #s first)*

1. _____

2. _____

3. _____

4. _____

5. _____

6. _____

7. _____

8. _____

9. _____

10. _____

11. Shavasana relaxation—don't forget to end with relaxation!

The best yoga teacher for your two-year-old can be you! Your preschooler is a great imitator. This is when your yoga practice becomes important, because a two-, three-, or four-year-old can learn or continue with yoga by mimicking you doing basic, simple yoga poses or any from the healthy yoga series you just created. It's time to strengthen your yoga practice and enjoy its benefits too!

Try incorporating your child's favorite animals or characters into yoga postures. Kids can pretend to be a horse, a bunny, a lion, a cat, a dog, or anything else they wish. Make sure yoga with your preschooler is full of animation and creative expression through movement. For example, if Halloween is approaching, teach yoga poses loosely based on what the child is dressing up as.

Have fun!

Finally, if you take class with a Certified Itsy Bitsy Yoga facilitator, he or she would be happy to recommend a yoga teacher for older children near you. Also, you can visit the resource websites listed below to find a qualified yoga teacher who has training, experience, and passion for teaching yoga to children.

Appendix

· · · · · · · · · · · ·

Resources:

www.baby-yoga.com
www.childrensyoga.com
www.itsybitsyyoga.com
www.nextgenerationyoga.com
www.specialyoga.com
www.yogakids.com

Developmental Play Poses

Sleep Well Poses

Tummy Time Poses